Getting the Best From Your Doctor

WITHDRAWN

An Insider's Guide to the Health Care You Deserve

Alan N. Schwartz, M.D.

Richard Jimenez, M.D.

Tracy Myers, M.H.A

Andrew Solomon, M.D.

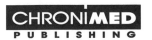
CHRONIMED PUBLISHING

Getting the Best From Your Doctor © 1998 by Alan N. Schwartz, Richard A. H. Jimenez, Tracy A. Myers, and Andrew K. Solomon

Library of Congress Cataloging-in-Publication Data

Schwartz, Alan N.

Getting the best from your doctor / by Alan N. Schwartz, Richard A. H. Jimenez, Tracy A. Myers, and Andrew K. Solomon

      p.   cm.

Includes index.

ISBN 1–56561–155–1; $23.95 ($33.95 Can.)

Acquiring Editor: Jeff Braun
Design & Production: David Enyeart
Art/Production Manager: Claire Lewis

Printed in the United States of America

Published by
Chronimed Publishing
P.O. Box 59032
Minneapolis, MN 55459-0032

10   9   8   7   6   5   4   3   2   1

Notice: Consult a Health Care Professional Because individual cases and needs vary, readers are advised to seek the guidance of a licensed physician, registered dietitian, or other health care professional before making changes in their prescribed health care regimens. This book is intended for informational purposes only and is not for use as an alternative to appropriate medical care. While every effort has been made to ensure that the information is the most current available, new research findings, being released with increasing frequency, may invalidate some data.

Stories included depict real events, but the names have been changed to protect individual identities.

WE WOULD LIKE TO ACKNOWLEDGE AND THANK:

Liz Dunne—whose encouragement and transcription of the original manuscript helped us greatly in our early efforts

Shannon Brownlee—whose ability to make words sparkle helped us get our book proposal accepted

Jeff Braun—whose editorial insight and skill transformed possibility into reality

Chronimed Publishing—whose mission to educate, serve, and empower patients is manifest in their publication of this book

Dr. Terrance R. McGuire and Dr. Taibi Kahler—whose lessons on Process Communication were the foundation for Chapter 2, "Do You Like Your Doctor?".

Mary Stadler, Marcia Houdek Jimenez, Kirsten Reinbold, and Bob Myers—whose loving support and constructive ideas were instrumental in improving the quality of this book

Dr. Richard Tonino, Dr. Marc Lerner, Dr. Malcolm Friedman, Jennifer Henriksen, Dr. Howard Uman, Jackie Delecki-Uman, Dr. Michael Norden, Dr. David Haynor, Dr. Jan Haynor, Dr. Bob Dalley, Dr. John Sylvester, Debby Stinson, Bob Schwartz, and Anamaria Lloyd—whose thoughts and opinions were greatly valued

Introduction

It's no secret that the world of health care is changing. Insurance policies are more restrictive than ever. Hospitals and managed care organizations are measuring the productivity of their staff. Doctors are being asked to be gatekeepers with a vested interest in not referring patients to specialists or ordering certain tests.

These changes are not just irritating. They can be dangerous to your health. If you are concerned about the current state of health care, from our vantage point, those concerns are justified. Our viewpoint is that of three physicians and a health care finance analyst. Unfortunately, what we are seeing are changes that are endangering lives and damaging the patient/doctor relationship, the heart of medicine. These disturbing observations and the knowledge that there is a remedy to these problems is what compelled us to write this book.

What's the remedy? Become your own best patient advocate. Now, more than ever, you and your family need to be well educated about your health. You need to communicate your medical needs clearly and effectively. And you need to be vigilant and know your rights.

Navigating the medical maze can feel overwhelming. *Getting the Best From Your Doctor* is an insider's perspective designed to show you where to start and how to proceed during difficult times. We can coach you on how to work effectively with your doctor and avoid many of the barriers and pitfalls imposed by the medical insurance and management industry. You will be able to take charge of your treatment and optimize your care rather than remaining a "passive sufferer"—the origin of the word *patient*. From learning how to communicate with your doctor to integrating the best of traditional and alternative medicine to creating your own medical miracles, this book will help you help yourself.

As frustrating as health care is nowadays, it is important to remember that you have a great deal of responsibility in your own care. An effective patient/doctor relationship is a partnership in which both individuals are engaged in a sort of dance. Each is looking to the other for information and feedback; each takes turns leading and following; each wants the treatment to be successful, balancing pain and risks against potential benefits.

Your doctor is your ally, not your adversary. Most physicians and health professionals have your best interests in mind. Still, doctors do make mistakes. Some do not communicate well with patients and some are serving their second master, their corporation and insurance company, rather than their first master—you, the patient.

Getting the Best From Your Doctor is organized in five sections, with each chapter representing a stage of the medical journey. We start by exploring the importance of effective communication—the basis of all good relationships, health-related or not. Then we present vital information about how to get organized for medical appointments. The book's third section is devoted to the different aspects of obtaining excellent care, from the medical test stage to prognosis. Next, we reveal what you should know about managed care systems and insurance coverage. And finally, we wrap up everything by covering your medical rights. Every chapter begins with a story about a patient, which expresses the chapter's theme. The body of the chapter presents the knowledge needed to improve your care. And the chapter ends with an interactive exercise or exercises to help you personalize the information. The value of this format is that you can choose to read the entire book or just focus on those chapters or exercise that satisfy your immediate and essential needs.

Getting the Best From Your Doctor provides you with the information and insights you need to become your own best patient advocate and receive the health care that you and your family deserve.

What's Your Health IQ?

The more "No" answers, the more you need to learn to get the health care you deserve.

When a doctor uses SOAP, do you know what that means?　Y　N

When you explain your medical problems to your doctor,
　do you know how to get him or her to really listen to you? Y　N

Do you know how to optimize your time with your doctor?　Y　N

Do you like your doctor?　Y　N

Do you know your doctor's personality style and does that
　style match yours?　Y　N

Do you know the four Principles of the Hippocratic Code?　Y　N

Do you know how to assess if your doctor is competent?　Y　N

Do you know when it's appropriate to seek a second opinion? Y　N

Do you know if your insurance company will pay for a
　second opinion?　Y　N

Can you do a medical information search on the Internet?　Y　N

Do you know the difference between a doctor's and a
　patient's definition of normal health?　Y　N

Are you capable of determining which medical symptoms
　may be dangerous to your health and survival?　Y　N

Do you practice preventive medicine?　Y　N

Do you know how to find the correct specialist to treat
　your illness?　Y　N

Do you know how to assess your doctor's qualifications?　Y　N

Do you know how to contact a doctor if you are out of town? Y　N

Do you know the difference between an otolaryngologist
　and an rheumatologist?　Y　N

Do you know when it is necessary to obtain prior autho-
　rization from your insurance company for medical care?　Y　N

Do you know how to organize, prepare, and prioritize
　your medical history and records?　Y　N

Do you know the difference between a chief complaint,
　a sign, and a symptom?　Y　N

Do you know how to obtain your past medical records　Y　N

Do you know that some of your medical records can be
　destroyed without your permission? Do you know how
　to have them preserved?　Y　N

Do you know the difference between the working, differential, and final diagnosis?	Y	N
Do you keep a medical log? Do you know what to record?	Y	N
Can you explain the difference between a routine, a specialized, and an experimental test?	Y	N
Do you know what to do if your doctor is unable to make an accurate diagnosis?	Y	N
Have you considered the advantages and disadvantages of traditional, alternative, and integrated medicine?	Y	N
Do you understand the term *integrated medicine?*	Y	N
Do you know how to measure the effectiveness of your treatment plan?	Y	N
Can you recognize when you are receiving sub-optimal care?	Y	N
Do you know what to do if your initial treatment fails?	Y	N
Have you ever considered the importance and the healing powers of faith and a positive attitude?	Y	N
Do you know what to do if your doctor is "stealing your hope"?	Y	N
Do you know what placebo is and how it influences the healing process?	Y	N
Do you know the difference between an HMO and a PPO?	Y	N
Do you know if there is a maximum lifetime benefit for your insurance plan?	Y	N
Do you know if your doctor works in a managed care program?	Y	N
Do you know how your gatekeeper is paid and how he or she earns bonuses?	Y	N
Do you know the difference between co-insurance and co-payment?	Y	N
Do you know that you can get transitional COBRA insurance if you change jobs?	Y	N
Do you know how to resolve a medical bill dispute?	Y	N
Do you have a living will?	Y	N
Do you know how to determine if a medical research study is safe for you?	Y	N
Are you familiar with the Patients' Bill of Rights?	Y	N

Score: Count up the number of "yes" and "no" answers ____ ____

A perfect health IQ is 50 "yes" answers.

Chapter 1

Poor Communication

The Curable Disease

At age 75, Martha Davis had a ruptured appendix. Both she and her doctors were surprised because a rupture of the appendix rarely occurs at that age. Her doctors puzzled over her case until they received a report from the pathologist. Under the microscope, a sample of tissue taken from her appendix during surgery revealed a cluster of cancerous tumor cells. A tumor is one of the few conditions known to cause a ruptured appendix in the elderly.

In order to determine the appropriate treatment, the doctors discussed the 'Davis Case' among themselves. They knew the cluster of tumor cells had been completely removed at surgery. Still, there was the unlikely but theoretical possibility that when the appendix burst some cancer cells may have spilled onto the lining of the abdomen. Because some of those malignant cells might not have been removed at the time of surgery, her physicians after much debate decided it would be best if Mrs. Davis received aggressive treatment. When they presented their treatment plan they simply told Mrs. Davis that she should undergo chemotherapy and radiation. They did not explain *how* they arrived at their treatment decision nor did they reveal their colleagues' misgivings about such aggressive therapy.

Behind closed doors, Mrs. Davis and her family privately questioned the doctor's aggressive recommendations and asked for additional studies to determine whether there was any evidence that cancer was still present in her body. The tests revealed no tumor.

Mrs. Davis respected her doctors but she was still uncomfortable with their advice. She and her family believed that chemotherapy and radiation were excessive. After all, she was 75 years old; the tumor had been completely removed and the side effects of treatment would be uncomfortable and possibly dangerous.

Mrs. Davis and her family agonized over all the information. Finally, she informed her doctors that she did not want the aggressive treatment; she would rather wait and see if the cancer reappeared. To her surprise, her doctors agreed with her. They said they had felt obligated to offer her the most aggressive approach, despite the fact that they didn't really think the cancer would likely recur. The family felt frustrated and wondered why the doctors hadn't just told them that in the first place.

This true story underscores how difficult it can be for doctors and patients to communicate. The doctors among themselves considered all available treatment options but they never communicated any of that decision-making process to the patient or her family. They never explained HOW they decided to recommend aggressive therapy. Mrs. Davis, who from the onset was uncomfortable with the proposed care, failed to express her dismay directly to the doctors and never asked for an explanation as to WHY aggressive chemotherapy and radiation were necessary. There was incomplete communication on both sides, and both parties could have done better.

Communication is indeed a two-way street. If you can change the way you communicate with your doctor, it will in turn change the way your doctor communicates and cares for you. Communication is one of the best ways, if not the best way, for patients to influence their care. But patients are often reluctant to take an active role and responsibility for their part in patient/doctor communication.

The word *patient* comes from the Greek word *pathos,* which means suffering. And for centuries, patients have literally been passive sufferers, obeying their doctors without question. The belief that the doctor is the expert with all the answers disempowers the patient and perpetuates the role of passive sufferer. In turn, this passive attitude of patients often interferes with the doctor's ability to deliver quality care. Your doctor can never know precisely what you are feeling; nor can he or she understand all the complex changes that are occurring in your health and body day-to-day unless you communicate that information. While the doctor has more knowledge of your disease initially, you and your family can educate yourselves so that you can become experts in your disease. By effectively communicating, you assist your doctor in the process of caring for you and your family.

Although this chapter is written primarily for the patient, it is our hope that doctors and health care providers will also be drawn to this information in order to better understand the relationship between patient and care giver. In the meantime, there are steps you can take today, as a patient, to begin improving communication with your care giver. We start by exploring how and why doctors communicate the way they do.

HOW COME MY DOCTOR CAN DO BRAIN SURGERY, BUT HE DOESN'T KNOW HOW TALK TO ME?

The answer is simple. Your doctor has been trained to be a doctor (to do brain surgery), but he has not necessarily been taught how to communicate effectively. He may not know the first thing about how to talk to patients because nobody ever taught him. Students are selected for medical school because of their scientific interests and abilities, not because of communication skills or teaching abilities. These communication skills are underemphasized in medical school. Instead, medical students learn how to diagnose and cure disease. They may never learn how to convey information to the patient.

So what can you, the patient, do to improve communication? You are 50 percent of the process. By improving your communication skills, your doctor might very well improve the way he communicates with you.

DOCTORSPEAK

If you've been to a doctor, you've heard DoctorSpeak: You come in complaining of an itch, and your doctor says you have *puritus*. That lump on your foot you call a bunion gets the tongue-twisting name *hallux valgus-metatarsus adductus*. DoctorSpeak is a medical foreign language. Every area of science, from anthropology to zoology, has its own specialized language or jargon. Medicine is no different. DoctorSpeak is the specialized language doctors use to talk to each other. Unfortunately, it is often the way they talk to their patients, as well.

How did DoctorSpeak develop? Hippocrates, the father of western medicine, was a Greek physician who lived around 400 B.C. His writings formed the basis for those who studied medicine after him. Following the Greeks, the Romans ruled the world and Latin became the official language of medicine and science. Since then, medical terminology has remained rooted in these Greek and Latin basics. Beginning in medical school, doctors are required to master and use these scientific terms in order to communicate with each other. There are advantages and disadvantages to using DoctorSpeak.

Medical terms are extremely specific, and serve as a shorthand, which allows doctors to communicate precisely with each other. This is particularly important when reading and writing scientific reports and papers; technical terms can save an entire explanatory paragraph.

Medical terms briefly and accurately detail an ailment and its location in the body. For example, the patient has a squamous cell carcinoma of the lingula. Translated, this refers to a specific type of cancer originating from the tissue in the front lower half of the left lung. You can see how much more efficient it is for doctors to use medical language when talking or writing to each other. DoctorSpeak gives physicians the ability to efficiently present and discuss complex concepts. Other common language terms are less precise and just do not convey the same meaning.

DoctorSpeak can be used as a secret fraternal handshake. It allows doctors to communicate only with a specific group of people while leaving others out of the conversation. It gives physicians a professional air or an aloofness, which sometimes can be interpreted as being pompous.

Doctors also use this specialized language to protect their emotions. Since doctors deal with a considerable amount of human misery and suffering, DoctorSpeak can be used to depersonalize a conversation. Sad and unpleasant events can be talked about in a detached and emotionless way. It is much easier to talk about "the lesion" than it is to talk about the brain tumor from which Ms. Jones is dying.

What may be advantageous to the doctor may be a disadvantage to the patient. DoctorSpeak can be used to talk *at* a patient without really communicating *with* the patient. This allows the doctor not only to protect her emotions, but also to hide them from her patient. Some doctors are uncomfortable confronting the sadness that comes with honestly facing another person's misery. The problem is, when doctors' emotions are hidden behind DoctorSpeak, it can sometimes be more difficult for patients to make "good" decisions concerning their care.

Should everyone take a Berlitz course in DoctorSpeak or hire a translator to accompany them each time they visit the doctor's office? No. Ideally, your doctor should be your translator. She should use the technical terms that are needed to be precise, but then translate those terms into everyday language. If she does not do this, then you may need to specifically ask her to speak in plain English.

REMEDY Ask your doctor to write out a summary of the conversation including any technical terms or complex concepts. Then you can look up the terms and concepts when you leave the office. If you would like more than a summary, ask your doctor if you can tape record the conversation so that you and your family can listen to it later.

INSIDER'S HINT

Ask the doctor to pretend that she is explaining your problem to her mother (assuming her mother is not a physician).

PATIENTSPEAK

A patient's language can be the antithesis of DoctorSpeak. PatientSpeak is filled with drama and emotions. Patients often speak in the language of illness, suffering, and pain. PatientSpeak deals almost exclusively with the patient and their immediate family. It is very much a personal language that reflects your perspective and feelings about your situation.

REMEDY To be effective communicators, we believe patients need to express not only their feelings but also the facts concerning their health.

COMMUNICATING USING SOAP

Doctors gather information from their patients by "taking a history"—a stylized format for recording an encounter with a patient that was popularized in the 1970s. Today, this format has been adopted by most physicians because it helps organize their approach to a patient's problem. The acronym for this approach is SOAP, which stands for:

S Subjective patient complaints.

O Objective findings on physical exam and diagnostic tests.

A Assessment of the illness, the diagnosis, and the prognosis.

P Plan for further evaluation and treatment.

The SOAP system works well for doctors because doctors have common objectives, with common reference points, which are communicated in a common language. The weakness in the SOAP system lies with S and O, the subjective and objective reporting of a medical problem. All too often, patients are not skilled in describing their concerns objectively and doctors are unable to elicit and understand their patient's subjective complaints.

A NEW METHOD OF COMMUNICATING WITH YOUR DOCTOR

To help you better communicate your illness, we suggest following a new system we call HOPE. This communication system focuses more on the patient's subjective feelings and needs, as well as delivering the objective facts. Here's what HOPE stands for:

- **H HISTORICAL FACTS:** Your objective reporting of what you have observed
- **O OPINIONS AND FEELINGS:** Your interpretation of the facts and their effects on you
- **P PERSONAL FEARS:** The worries that have been created by your illness
- **E EXPECTATIONS AND REQUESTS:** Your desires for the evaluation and treatment

The goal of this system is to let the patient better express both emotions and facts, in an order and format that will be more palatable to most doctors. By presenting information in this manner, the doctor will better understand your medical problems and concerns, and will be more responsive.

Let's go through an example of how HOPE can be used to improve a patient/physician encounter. Below are two extremes of patient approaches drawn from real experiences.

THE ANGRY PATIENT: "Doctor, I don't think your treatment is doing me any good. I am in pain and nervous all the time. I'm worried I'm going to die. Nothing you prescribe works, and I am afraid that I may lose my job because of this stupid ulcer. I know I have an ulcer. You know I have an ulcer. So why can't you just fix it, now! I know you came highly recommended, but you're not helping me. If you can't handle this problem I'll find someone else that can. So what are you going to do about this?"

The angry patient is frightened and feels out of control, but instead of appealing to the doctor for help, he lashes out in fear. The less enlightened doctor tunes out such patients. Some doctors may even tell angry patients to find their medical care someplace else—a response doctors refer to privately as "firing" a patient. Other doctors may lose all empathy for the patient, though they will continue treating his ailment.

THE PATIENT WHO WANTS TO PLEASE THE DOCTOR: "Doctor, do you think I'm getting better? I still have some pain, but I think you're a good doctor and doing a good job."

This patient also feels fearful but cannot express the problem. Instead, he makes statements that mislead the doctor into assuming the patient is improving on the current regimen of treatment. The patient, in turn, continues to have pain and grows more fearful. The two may circle each other in this dance of misunderstanding until a critical point is reached. Either the patient's condition deteriorates, the doctor figures out all is not well, the patient's spouse calls with concerns, or the patient sees a new doctor.

COMMUNICATING USING HOPE

Variations on these examples occur regularly, and both are non-productive in different ways. The better approach for communicating with your doctor is the HOPE method:

You are experiencing stomach pain and you go to your doctor for an evaluation. You report the:

H HISTORICAL FACTS, RELATING TO YOUR SYMPTOMS: "Doctor, I've got recurring pain in my stomach. It starts 10 minutes after I eat. Spicy foods and stress seem to make it worse. Antacids help sometimes, but only for a short time."

O OPINION AND FEELINGS: "I feel awful and the pain is making me irritable. I can't eat or do the things I enjoy. I think I'm getting worse."

P PERSONAL FEARS: "I'm afraid that I have a bleeding ulcer and that I could die from it. My Uncle Ned almost died from a bleeding ulcer."

E EXPECTATIONS AND REQUESTS: "I like you and want to keep you as my doctor, but I need some relief soon. I'd like either a stronger medicine or some tests to find out whether I have a bleeding ulcer."

Your doctor may not meet your expectations or grant your requests. However, he will have a clear understanding of your symptoms and how they affect you, both physically and emotionally. He will know what issues need to be discussed, and he should address your expectations. You will help your doctor by separating the factual content of the information from the emotional content and by clearly stating your expectations. This provides a strong foundation for the rest of your communications. Exercise 1-1 will help you to organize your HOPE approach.

INSIDER'S HINT
....
To get help, communicate with HOPE.

CAN YOU BE A CREDIBLE WITNESS?

Hand-in-hand with presenting your problem to a doctor in an organized manner is the vital concept of credibility. All too often, patients ask, "Why doesn't my doctor believe me?" and "How can I get my doctor to believe me?" This frustration with patient/doctor communication is based on two factors.

First, doctors are trained to be skeptical and critical. They learn and memorize many facts, but they are also taught how to analyze and interpret them. This applies not only to scientific articles but to evaluating a patient's illness. Many doctors will not believe another doctor's diagnosis until they have examined the patient themselves and verified all the test results. This approach is a great benefit to the patient. It helps to ensure that the doctor's opinions and decisions are his own and that he stands behind his recommended treatment.

This training, however, also leads the doctor to question everything the patient says. If the doctor cannot verify something that the patient describes, then his training leads him to doubt its accuracy.

The second factor related to the question of credibility is that most patients are not trained in communication either. Many people describe their ailments through a disjointed, rambling story loaded with emotional editorial comments that are hard for doctors to understand. Symptoms, illnesses, and treatments are often described incompletely and inadequately. A doctor who is trained to analyze facts critically can end up not believing much of what a patient says.

To paraphrase Sir Isaac Newton, "Every exaggeration has an equal and opposite reaction." That is to say, the more a patient exaggerates his symptoms, the less his doctor is inclined to believe the story—

even if it has very real elements of truth. The same story told in an emotional but accurate manner causes the doctor to want to reach out and help the patient, both emotionally and medically.

HOW DO YOU GET YOUR DOCTOR TO BELIEVE YOU?

This can be a very hard task, especially if your symptoms are ill-defined or unusual. Our best advice is to be a good witness and tell the truth—and nothing but the truth—about your condition.

FIRST, BE ACCURATE. Try not to minimize or exaggerate your symptoms. This will only mislead your doctor and may delay your care. Some people embellish facts because they think doctors only listen if it sounds serious. Dramatization seldom works and understating symptoms can lead to delays in diagnosis and treatment.

TRY NOT TO DESCRIBE YOUR SYMPTOMS WITH SUPERLATIVES, SUCH AS HORRENDOUS COUGH, OR EXCRUCIATING PAIN. Rather, it is best to take a lesson from DoctorSpeak and grade the symptoms as mild, moderate, and severe. If one symptom is worse than another, save the superlatives for that particular symptom. Use terms that are based on the five senses. Describe what you see, hear, feel, taste and smell.

Some patients are pegged as hypochondriacs because they see their doctor for every minor complaint. They read about a disease and are suddenly convinced they have that illness. This Boy-That-Cried-Wolf situation can lead doctors to doubt a patient's veracity even when the patient has legitimate concerns.

IT IS ALSO NOT FAIR TO GO INTO THE DOCTOR'S OFFICE WITH A HIDDEN AGENDA. Some people practically challenge their doctor to figure out what is wrong. Don't try to find out how smart your doctor really is by withholding information about your symptoms and forcing her to guess. Instead, show that you want to work with her to get better results.

IMMEDIATELY ASKING YOUR DOCTOR FOR STRONG NARCOTICS OR OTHER ADDICTIVE DRUGS, PARTICULARLY ON YOUR FIRST VISIT, WILL PROBABLY ONLY RAISE SUSPICIONS THAT YOUR SYMPTOMS ARE FICTITIOUS. You may be viewed as a liar. Doctors do encounter drug seekers or drug dealers who come into the office with the expressed purpose of acquiring drugs to treat their habit or to resell the medications illegally. However, once your illness is understood by your doctor, the same request for narcotics or stronger pain killers may be appropriate if the pain is not controlled by the medications prescribed.

No matter what, try to present a concise, streamlined, cogent description of your illness. Model yourself as a good witness, one who would be believed by a jury of your peers. In order for your symptoms to be believable to your doctor, they must be well presented and seem within the realm of possibility. Even dubious stories can be made believable if presented properly. Exercise 1-2 will help you to determine if there is some reason your doctor might question your credibility.

To make sure your doctor will believe you,

Do:
Be accurate

Be honest

Be direct

Be prepared

Be courteous and friendly

Be subjective in your feelings

Be objective in your
   observation

Don't:
Don't exaggerate or minimize
   symptoms

Don't lie

Don't play games

Don't expect a miracle

Don't come in with a hidden
   agenda

Don't be afraid to express your
   opinions

Don't ask for narcotics on the
   first visit

Don't take out your frustrations
   on your doctor

Don't conceal your emotions,
   but don't let them run wild

PatientListen (Active Patient Listening)

To paraphrase Oscar Wilde, "Doctors and patients are separated by a common language." There is often a dichotomy between what one person says, and means, and what the other person hears, or understands. Just as several eyewitnesses can observe a single event and reach different conclusions, patients and physicians can walk away from the examining room with different perspectives about what transpired. Here's an example.

A young woman, we'll call her Jane Smith, gave birth to a 7½ pound girl, who seemed perfectly healthy at delivery. But her pediatrician noticed several subtle birth defects, including too many skin folds about the neck, puffy hands and feet, and perfectly spiraling fingerprints. A genetic counselor, we'll call him Dr. Black, was called in to evaluate Baby Girl Smith, and he ordered several tests. A week later, the Smiths visited Dr. Black in his office to discuss the results of his investigations.

Dr. Black told the Smiths their baby had Turner's Syndrome, a genetic abnormality that would cause their daughter to be shorter in stature than normal, unable to have children, and likely have cosmetic defects and learning disabilities. After telling the Smiths this news, Dr. Black paused and asked them if they had understood what he said, and if they had any questions. They said they understood and had no questions.

Dr. Black continued to talk for another 30 minutes, explaining the many challenges the Smiths would face in the upcoming years. At the end of his discussion, he gave them a prepared synopsis of what he had discussed. He asked them to read it and sign a signature sheet acknowledging that they had understood what they had just read. He also asked them to write in the chart in their own words what they had just learned. They did so and signed their note.

One year later, the Smiths returned to the hospital for a follow-up genetics appointment. They were scheduled to see Dr. Black, who in the interim had changed his appearance by shedding his long hair, growing a mustache, and adopting a more conservative style of dress. They didn't recognize him when they walked into his office. They introduced themselves and began telling Dr. Black how little they understood about their child's condition. They said the genetic counselor they saw just after their daughter's birth had been very nice, but he had not given them much information. Dr. Black smiled and asked them if they remembered which doctor they had seen.

They did not remember. Dr. Black revealed that he was their genetic counselor. He opened their daughter's chart and showed them the synopsis they had read and signed, as well as the summary of the counseling session that they had written in their own words.

The Smiths were visibly embarrassed. They did not remember any of that information communicated at that first visit, but there it was in their own writing. They did remember, however, how distraught they were after hearing the news about their daughter. A year had gone by, and now they were prepared to listen. They were now attentive, and at the end of the session, they were grateful for the information and the understanding manner in which Dr. Black communicated that information.

This real example demonstrates that even if a physician takes a great deal of care to discuss a medical problem with empathy, the patient may not hear or understand the information if it is presented during emotionally charged moments. It is valuable for both doctors and patients to realize that communication is only successful if the message received is the same as the message expressed.

By asking your doctor probing questions you can help ensure that the message received is the same as the message sent. It is vital to make sure you understand what your doctor is saying; discuss your illness a second time, after your peak emotions have subsided. This can be accomplished through repetition of information, during follow-up appointments, and by insisting that there is an intelligent simplicity to the doctor's explanations and information.

Studies show that people remember only a fraction of what their doctors have told them 10 minutes after they leave the office. There are several reasons for this. As in the previous story, your emotions may take over after hearing a disturbing diagnosis. If your doctor says, "You have cancer of the breast," you may not hear another word. In fact, while the diagnosis is conjuring images and fears about future surgery and pain, you might not hear your doctor say, "Fortunately, it's a very tiny tumor that can be removed with a lumpectomy." Sometimes the sheer volumes of information a doctor must convey overwhelms your ability to take it all in at once.

Some patients miss important details and facts because they are not paying strict attention. They are thinking about their next appointment or getting back to work. Some people don't want the details, they are only interested in the "diagnostic punch line." Others may be anxious for a prescription so that they can walk out the door, fill it, and start on the road to getting well.

As we said before, communication is a two-way street. If you can change the way you communicate with your doctor, it will in turn change the way your doctor communicates and cares for you. If you bridge the communication gap, you will empower your relationship and optimize your chances for wellness. Becoming active in the communication process begins with developing a common communication style.

Finally, it is important to remember to separate the message from the messenger. The doctor didn't make you sick (in most cases), but he is trying to make you better. Don't shoot the messenger. Ask him for his help. Don't let fears, ego, or pride get in the way of getting healthy.

We believe you can improve your PatientListening by applying Active Patient Listening:

KEYS TO ACTIVE PATIENT LISTENING

FOCUSED LISTENING

- Concentrate on what is being said.
- Provide yourself with enough time so that you do not feel rushed.
- Try not to have any distractions, such as young children, in the exam room, so that you can give your undivided attention.
- Quiet your internal thoughts and fears so that you can hear and receive the doctor's message.

WRITTEN LISTENING

- This is essentially note taking. Write down the essential points you want to remember.
- Consider asking the doctor to write down the diagnosis, treatment plan, and prescriptions.

WITNESSED LISTENING

- You may feel highly emotional and unable to concentrate on the details. If that is the situation, try to have a relative or friend with you to listen to the explanation.

ECHOED LISTENING

- Restate in common language what you think the doctor has said to you. You may be surprised to find that what you hear differs from what has been said.

COURAGEOUS LISTENING

- Do not pretend that you understand if you do not. Ask questions or have your witness ask questions until you feel you understand what the doctor has said.
- Try not to be afraid to hear the truth. The truth may be less frightening than your imagination or denial. If your reality is frightening, the best way to confront it is with truth, courage, and strength.
- No one can understand and remember 100 percent of what the doctor tells them. The goal is to remember the information that you need to remember.

MANAGING YOUR TIME WITH YOUR DOCTOR

Most patients want more time to discuss their situation. Doctors, however, have limited amounts of time to spend with you. Office visits are scheduled for a certain amount of time, depending on the expected complexity of your problems. A new patient office visit may be anywhere from 30 to 60 minutes. Return visits are usually between 10 and 30 minutes. In Chapter 9 we discuss the time management of an office visit.

Doctors want you to get better and would like to spend as much time as necessary to help you do this. The reality, however, is that good doctors are very busy with many patients wanting to be seen. Doctors who are employees of a health maintenance organization (HMO) or other organization may even be told how much time to spend with each patient. If this time limit is exceeded by even a modest amount, it can have repercussions throughout the day and may result in all subsequent patients getting less time with the doctor.

The key is to optimize your time with your doctor. Prepare, organize, and prioritize your needs (Chapters 7 and 8) so that you can efficiently use your time with the doctor. If you have seven concerns you would like to discuss and only have 15 to 20 minutes, it is unlikely that anything will be addressed adequately unless you are organized, prepared, and willing to voice only your most pressing concerns.

INSIDER'S HINT

Prescription for Effective Patient Communication:
Preparation—Organization—Prioritization

DOCTORLISTEN (EFFECTIVE DOCTOR LISTENING)

For some doctors, bedside manner comes naturally. But for most doctors, good communication is like playing a musical instrument; it must be learned and then practiced to be perfected. The best physician communicators have an open mind, a receptive ear, and an empathic heart. Their good bedside manner is perfected through practice, experience, and feedback from patients and other doctors.

For communication to be effective, the doctor must be attuned to your communication style. Different people need different forms of communication from their doctor. Some patients require emotional dialogue, for example. They want a doctor who lays her hand on their arm and says, "You're looking great. How are you feeling?" Another patient might be more comfortable with a more analytical approach and a doctor who sits back in his chair and says, "Your numbers look good." The difference in doctors' styles is important but often under appreciated.

You can optimize your chance for successful communication by choosing a doctor that fits your style. In Chapter 2 we discuss how you can determine both your style as well as that of your doctor.

If you happen to choose a doctor who does not perfectly match your style, you may need to help your doctor understand your needs by providing both positive and negative feedback. Tell your doctor you don't understand the technical terms, or use the "P" (Personal Fears) in HOPE to help your doctor understand your fears and frustration.

How well your doctor communicates is influenced by a number of factors. Is the doctor comfortable with the message he is about to deliver? Is the doctor comfortable discussing that particular illness? Does the doctor tell the patient everything about the illness in one session? Does the doctor tell the patient the heart truth—information conveyed with empathy and understanding—or merely the hard truth—information told in a factual and technically precise manner with no empathy? Communication is effective if the message is accurately received. To accomplish this the message should be easily understood and the messenger empathetic enough to perceive the needs of the listener.

To improve communication, especially with a potentially serious illness, you might want to tell your doctor how much information you are prepared to hear. It helps doctors if a patient says, "I want to know what I have. Please be honest with me. I would rather know what I have than to continue not knowing. Please tell me the whole truth." Another patient might say, "Can I discuss the details at a second visit with my spouse present? I don't think I am prepared to hear any more today."

Finally, it is important for patients and doctors to focus on each other. This may seem like common sense, but you would be surprised how often patients and doctors come into the exam room and seem in a hurry or distracted. You and your doctor should be seated and looking directly at each other. Focus on each other, not the chart, the x-ray films, or the view out the window. Give each other the attention and respect the situation deserves.

WHAT CAN YOU DO TODAY TO HELP YOUR DOCTOR LISTEN MORE EFFECTIVELY?

Communication is more than just the words. Communication experts and psychologists estimate that 7 percent of any message is the spoken word, 38 percent is voice quality (tone of voice, tempo, intonation) and 55 percent is the body language that accompanies the spoken word. (We actually believe that the actual words spoken are powerful and account for more than 7% of the message.) Nevertheless, the message behind these statistics is that much of how we communicate is non-verbal. For a doctor to effectively understand his patient, he must be aware of the non-verbal cues. This involves first teaching doctors how to recognize non-verbal cues and, if the verbal and the non-verbal cues are mismatched, teaching the doctor how to learn the 'true' meaning of the patient's message.

For both patients and doctors, body language is very important. For instance, you probably feel a doctor is more interested and a better communicator if she sits rather than stands when talking to you. Sitting creates the feeling that the doctor is focusing on and taking time with you, not rushing off to her next appointment. Not surprisingly, if one doctor sits for 5 minutes while another stands for 10 minutes, more patients will believe that the seated doctor is more connected and caring toward them, even though he spent less time. Other forms of body language, such as an "open" stance, or touching, are important and have similar effects on patient-doctor communication. As the patient, if you feel rushed or you are made uncomfortable by your doctor, or if he paces or stands during the whole exam, observe his body language. Then, consider asking him to sit when he talks with you. When you are in the hospital this can be particularly important because you may be feeling especially vulnerable.

A doctor also needs to realize that his words will influence your understanding of the message. Explaining a diagnosis or treatment can improve a patient's understanding of the disease—which in turn can influence a patient's willingness to comply with treatment. But more words are not always more effective. Studies have looked at patients who were presented with either a long, detailed, and technical explanation of their treatment or a short, simplified, and non-technical explanation. Which do you think was better understood? The short, simplified, and non-technical version. In addition to remembering more information, patients felt that the doctor presenting the shorter version did a better job. If your doctor begins to get long winded and too technical, stop her and ask for the shortened *Reader's Digest* version. Just be sure to tell the doctor to include all the important details.

Voice quality has a powerful impact on your ability to hear the message accurately. Some patients want a warm, maternalistic or paternalistic tone. For other patients, this is an immediate turn-off; they prefer a cordial but less familiar approach. A hurried tone may be interpreted as evidence that the doctor doesn't care. A benign diagnosis delivered with serious undertones in a hurried manner may lead the patient to believe that her ailment is more serious than the doctor is letting on. If you are not comfortable with your doctor's tone, or if the words and tone are mismatched, stop your doctor and tell him. If he can't change, won't change, or gets insulted, perhaps you need to change doctors.

Is Your Doctor a Good Communicator?
- Does your doctor uses words and language that you can understand?
- Does your doctor's style matches your style enough to meet your needs?
- Does your doctor is clear about what he intends to accomplish with each visit?
- Does your doctor focuses his attention on you and your needs?

The 'How' and 'Why' of the Patient/Doctor Partnership

Health is a collaborative effort, one that requires the participation of both the patient and the doctor. To have a strong patient/doctor relationship both partners must be effective communicators. The doctors need to explain to their patients HOW they arrived at their diagnosis and treatment plan. In return, patients need to understand WHY it is so important that they follow the doctor's medical recommendations. Problems frequently arise when either partner fails to uphold their responsibility in communication. Without this partnership, doctors are often frustrated with their patient's unwillingness to follow instructions and accept their responsibility for returning to wellness. In turn, patients are frequently frustrated with their doctors because their doctors have failed to explain important information to them.

The key ingredient missing in such cases is communication. A patient with a herniated disc, which is a very serious injury to the back, is told by his doctor not to lift anything heavier than a pencil for two months. Three days later, the patient shows up in the emergency room because he tried to move his piano.

Defensively the patient explains, "But I felt better."

The frustrated doctor responds, "But I told you not to lift anything heavy for at least two months."

In this case both parties failed to do their part to foster communication. Although the doctor gave explicit instructions to the patient. The doctor did not help the patient understand the consequences— the WHY—of not following instructions. The patient, on the other hand, did not listen to or understand the importance of strictly complying with the doctors prescription of activity.

It is your doctor's job to know how to communicate with patients. But if the two of you are not communicating effectively, it is you, not the doctor, who will suffer the greatest consequences. Knowing SOAP and HOPE, being a credible witness, managing your time, and recognizing effective communication are the foundation to a good doctor-patient relationship.

But, there is more!

We recommend that you the patient take responsibility for effective communication. Communication is one of the few variables over which you have control. You may start out understanding very little about your disease, but with good communication and research you can become an informed participant in your decision making process.

Since poor communication is a curable disease, the side effects of poor communication can be minimized. If the dialogue is unclear, it is the your responsibility to ask and re-ask questions until the information is understandable. You may not have control over your disease or your physician's behavior, but you do have control over how you communicate.

INSIDER'S HINT

You have control over how you communicate. So…

Be proactive and take responsibility for promoting good communication.

Learn the goals of communication. You will help your doctor give you better care.

HOPE

To organize your time with the doctor, discuss your situation in the order as defined by the acronym HOPE. It stands for Historical facts, Opinions and feelings, Personal fears, and Expectations and requests.

HISTORICAL FACTS

First discuss the facts. If you start with the facts you will communicate to the physician in a way that he can assess your problem and treat your illness. Symptoms can be expressed in the form of an objective statement, such as:

Doctor, I have, _____

(describe objectively what you feel, see, smell, taste, and/or hear)

The_____ treatment helps _____

(specify treatment)   *(describe how it helps)*

But _____

(describe limitations of the treatment)

OPINIONS AND FEELINGS

Once the facts are out of the way, you can then concentrate on your opinions and feelings. Feelings and opinions can be expressed in emotional terms, such as:

I think _____

(describe analytic and objective thoughts)

I feel _____

(describe feelings and emotions)

I sense _____

(describe impressions and less well defined sensations)

EXERCISE 1-1

HOPE *(cont.)*

PERSONAL FEARS

It is important to discuss any fears you may have regarding your disease, your treatment, the accuracy of a diagnosis, side effects of medications, response of loved ones, and fears of your doctor's disapproval. Fears should be stated as clearly as possible. Fears may appear irrational or illogical, but don't worry about that. Expression of fears may take the form of statements or questions, such as:

I am afraid that _____

(describe specific past, present and/or future fears related to the illness)

EXPECTATIONS AND REQUESTS

Finally, ask for what you need. Discuss your expectations and any requests you may have with your doctor. By putting your needs into the form of a request, your doctor is obligated to address and, at least, attempt to deal with the request. Requests are usually in the form of:

I feel that I need _____

(describe your present needs)

I would like _____

(describe your solution to the problem)

AN EXAMPLE OF THE HOPE FORMAT

"**Doctor, I have** recurring pain in my stomach that begins 10 minutes after I eat. Spicy foods and stress seem to make it worse. The antacids (treatment) **help** sometimes, **but** only for a short time.

"**I feel** awful and the pain is making me irritable. I can't eat or do the things I enjoy. **I think** I am getting worse.

"**I am afraid** that I have a bleeding ulcer and that I could die from it. My uncle Ned almost died from a bleeding ulcer.

"**I feel that I need** some relief soon. **I would like** either a stronger medicine or some tests to find out whether or not I have a bleeding ulcer."

EXERCISE 1-2

A Credibility Check

Do you think your doctor doesn't believe you? Here are some questions to ask yourself, using your last encounter as a reference point.

1. Write out the information you presented to the doctor.

2. Does it make sense to you?

3. Does it make sense to your spouse or another trusted family member?

4. Were you (check the ones that apply to you):

___ Prepared	or	___ Unprepared
___ Courteous	or	___ Disrespectful
___ Honest	or	___ Evasive
___ Factual	or	___ Dramatic and Emotional
___ Consistent	or	___ Inconsistent
___ Requesting Help	or	___ Demanding Help

If some of your answers are in the second column, then you might have a credibility problem. Any of the characteristics in the second column could lead your doctor to question your reliability.

Chapter 2

Do You Like Your Doctor?

Shirley Ash was 76 when she was diagnosed with ovarian cancer. Her diagnosis came 10 days after her last friend in the world had died. With neither friends nor family to ease her suffering, Shirley underwent eight weeks of intensive chemotherapy. Despite her doctor's efforts, the cancer spread throughout her body. She grew more and more frail and gaunt.

John was a third year medical student when he met Shirley on the cancer ward, where she spent her days lying motionless in a dark room. In contrast to her morbid appearance, Shirley still had a lively wit and a spirited demeanor. John grew fond of her and visited her more often than any of his other patients.

John assumed that Shirley's private physician had put her in the hospital for aggressive chemotherapy at her own insistence. On the contrary, one day Shirley revealed that she felt she was dying and withstood the therapy only to "please her doctor and make him happy." One evening, when Shirley was looking and feeling particularly ill, John asked if there was anything she wanted before she died. Her face brightened and she answered, "I would love a manicure and perm so that I can look good for my friends in heaven."

The following day, the hospital staff raised the money for Shirley's makeover. A beautician came to the hospital that evening to wash and curl her few remaining strands of hair. She manicured Shirley's nails and massaged her withered hands. Afterward, Shirley beamed and said she once again felt human and very loved.

The next morning, John hurried to the ward to see Shirley, but she was dead. Later that day on rounds in front of all his fellow doctors, John was harshly criticized by the chief oncology resident for arranging the beautician for Shirley. The resident accused John of being overly sentimental and irresponsible instead of being a good doctor, searching for new ways to cure Shirley's disease.

This true story illustrates a crucial insight regarding the practice of medicine: For the most part, doctors are trained to attack diseases, not to necessarily care for the emotional needs of patients. Yet, sometimes, what is really best for the patient is for the doctor to listen and address the patient's emotional needs in order to reduce pain and suffering. Perhaps through a sense of being loved, Shirley Ash found the inner strength to die peacefully. For other patients who are less critically ill, this same feeling of being cared for—combined with good medical treatment—may work synergistically to bring about a cure.

THE ART OF MEDICINE

Medicine is an art that cannot be memorized. It must be learned through experience. As a result, each doctor delivers care and expresses the art of medicine in his or her own unique way. You will be best served by a doctor who is attuned and responds to both your medical and emotional needs—needs that vary from patient to patient, depending on the person's personality, life circumstances, and the severity and stage of illness.

- This chapter is devoted to helping you to determine if the doctor you have found is the right one for you.
- It will help you determine your own style, your doctor's style, and whether the two are well-matched.
- It will help you sort out your various (sometimes conflicting) feelings about your doctor.
- If there are communication problems between you and your doctor, this chapter will help you determine how they have developed, and, more importantly, how to solve the problem.

INSIDER'S HINT

A good relationship with your doctor is a powerful ally in the healing process.

WHAT CAN YOU EXPECT FROM YOUR DOCTOR/PHYSICIAN?

The term doctor is derived from the Latin word *docere*, which means to teach. The term physician takes its origin from the French word *fisique*, meaning the art of healing. In ancient cultures, doctors were thought to be men of great learning who possessed the powers to heal. The observation that we use the terms medical doctor and physician interchangeably suggests that we expect our health providers to be both teachers and healers. So, what should you expect from your doctor/physician?

A capable doctor should help teach you ways to:
• Maintain wellness through prevention
• Detect early signs of illness
• Understand when you should seek medical assistance
• Understand your illness and its treatment

The competent physician should also:
• Strive to make accurate diagnosis
• Prescribe the best treatment
• Work to relieve your physical pain and emotional suffering
• Monitor your progress and adjust treatments accordingly

EVALUATING YOUR DOCTOR'S PERFORMANCE

The Hippocratic Code provides a framework in which you can evaluate your doctor. Hippocrates was born approximately 460 B.C. on the Greek island of Cos. He is considered the father of Western Medicine. Of all his contributions, perhaps the most lasting and important is his Hippocratic Code (not to be confused with the Hippocratic Oath which it is believed he did not write). The Code outlines the principles by which a doctor should practice.

A summary of the four basic principals which your doctor should apply are:
1. Observe carefully
2. Know the patient at least as well as you know the disease
3. Evaluate honestly, accurately, and objectively
4. Assist nature or at least do no harm

These principles apply as much today as they did 2000 years ago and should form the basis of both how your doctor practices medicine and how you (the patient) evaluate your doctor.

What Is Your Gut Reaction? Everyone has gut reactions to the people they meet. Your reaction to your doctor is no exception. Some people make snap decisions about others based on their instincts, while others analyze the situation for days or weeks before deciding how they feel. Whatever your nature, it is important that you have a positive gut reaction about your doctor if you hope to optimize your chances for healing.

YOUR DOCTOR'S STYLE

Sometimes it helps to understand why you have a gut reaction to your doctor. Your doctor's style will strongly influence the way you feel about him or her, and it will influence how the two of you interact. Just like in Olympic figure skating, you must judge your doctor for both technical merit and artistic style. You will more likely award a 10 for your doctor's skills in the art of medicine if his or her style matches your needs.

To help you assess your doctor's style, we provide brief descriptions of the most common archetypes of doctors. (The system described below is based on a personality evaluation method used to choose the most qualified astronauts for the original Apollo and Gemini flights. This system called Process Communication was developed by Dr. Taibi Kahler and by Dr. Terrance F. McGuire.) Granted, we have narrowed these down to a few generalized styles, but for the most part they represent the vast majority of doctors. You should keep in mind that most doctors will be a combination of one or more styles, since all people have complex personalities. However, one style will usually dominate.

IS HE MARCUS WELBY?

If real life were like television, doctors would be as gentle and kind as Marcus Welby, patients would adore their doctors, and all diseases would be curable. But television rarely resembles life's harsher realities, and the myth of Marcus Welby is a stereotype that damages the doctor-patient relationship by creating unrealistic hopes and expectations.

Still, in real life there are some doctors who embody the traits admired in Marcus Welby. They are sensitive, compassionate, and comforting physicians. They focus on emotions. They usually have a good bedside manner and have the capacity to make you feel cared for.

Marcus Welby doctors can also become overly emotional and lose their objectivity when asked to impartially analyze an emotionally charged situation. For instance, if you disobey his instructions, a Marcus Welby may take it personally and feel wounded by your disobedience. Marcus Welby doctors can at times behave more as supportive cheerleaders than hard thinking analytic investigators for difficult to treat or diagnose illnesses. But when a Marcus Welby combines an empathetic ability with good analytic skills and native intelligence, he can comfort and guide you through even the most difficult illnesses and treatments.

IS HE MR. SPOCK?

This group comprises the largest subset of doctors. They are practical, analytical, and dedicated to their work and principles. Like Spock of the television series "Star Trek" (not to be confused with Dr. Spock, the late pediatrician), they concentrate on "the facts." These doctors are highly motivated, often workaholic physicians. They are concerned about you, but they may not show it emotionally. Instead, they work hard for you all hours, day and night. They often make work a priority above almost everything in their lives, including their own families. Their identity and ego is strongly tied to medicine. Don't expect hugs from this type. They care, but they may show it by going to the library or using the Internet to search the medical journals for answers to your health problems. Spock will be ethical and work hard for you.

IS SHE THE SCHOLARLY PROFESSOR?

These doctors are imaginative and creative. They are scholarly and sometimes appear to be "dancing to a different drummer." They are also among the most knowledgeable of doctors, and they are frequently found at universities doing medical research. They focus on solving complex problems that can both benefit humanity and advance the field of medicine.

You may need a scholarly professor for a second or expert opinion, since this type of doctor is often an expert in rare illnesses and difficult cases. Don't take it too personally if this doctor seems more comfortable with her lab rats or newest million-dollar medical technologic toy than with you, the patient. The scholarly professor will be a wonderful resource for difficult and complex medical problems.

IS HE A PERSUASIVE CHARMER?

Persuasive charmers are the rarest subset of doctors. They are often charismatic and flamboyant, and persuasive. (Eddie Haskel of "Leave It To Beaver" was a persuasive charmer.) They may have a stronger monetary focus and are more stylish and showy than other doctors. What works best for them is what is often uppermost in their minds. The persuasive charmer will be the doctor who commercializes new ideas for the medical marketplace (ideas usually created by the scholarly professor).

If you're not sure if your doctor is a persuasive charmer or just a very forceful person, ask yourself a few questions: Does he put style over substance? In other words, does it seem as if he puts his own needs—making money, for instance, or gathering prestige—above yours? Do you feel like he's trying to sell you something? If you go to a plastic surgeon for a facelift and he tries to sell you breast augmentation, you've probably found a persuasive charmer.

You should realize that many persuasive charmers are incredibly talented and capable physicians. If their objectives and goals match yours, then they can be of great benefit to you. A persuasive charmer who has her own clinic that is doing a booming business may be the perfect doctor to perform that facelift precisely because she has had a great deal of experience. At their best, persuasive charmers can bring new techniques into the marketplace and perform wonders.

Nevertheless, we caution you to investigate carefully doctors who are persuasive charmers. At their worst, they can be snake oil salesmen, trying to sell you unnecessary procedures or unproved therapies. Doctors pushing laetrile on cancer patients is a glaring example of this. Do your homework; ask other patients if this persuasive charmer is a doctor who can be trusted.

DOES YOUR DOCTOR FIT YOUR STYLE?

After you have made an attempt to classify your doctor's style, then it's time to ask, "What is my style?" Are you more of the analytical, emotional, scholarly, or charismatic type? What do you want from a doctor?

Matching your style with your doctor's style is critical to your ability to get the best care. If you are talkative and your doctor is quiet, you may walk away from an appointment feeling as if you did not get enough information. If you are an accountant who needs precision, details, and analysis, while your doctor is more touchy-feely and abstract, you may feel frustrated by your doctor's style. If there is a personality clash between the patient and the doctor, it doesn't necessarily mean that the doctor is bad—it may simply be a matter of a bad fit.

For example, several years ago Tonya Graham had been experiencing several unusual symptoms that her family physician could not diagnose, including joint pains, fatigue, and swollen legs. While watching a TV talk show, she learned that her symptoms might be due to a disease called lupus, and could even be related to her silicone breast implants. The next day she called the local lupus society and was given the name of Dr. Michaels, a local expert.

Though she saw Dr. Michaels for the next three years, she was never really comfortable with his personality. During appointments, they would discuss her symptoms and the possible causes for them. Then Dr. Michaels would lay out her treatment options. It was all very clear, and she believed he was giving her excellent care. But he never touched her, not to re-examine her, not to console her, not even to shake her hand when he said hello or good-bye. She trusted his medical judgment, but she realized there was something missing that she needed in order to feel comfortable and confident with Dr. Michaels' care. She ended up in another rheumatologist's waiting room, searching not for a second opinion but rather a doctor who would provide the missing ingredient, the personal human touch that she needed.

You need to think hard about what you really need and want from a doctor. Do you want a physician with a style that matches your style? Tonya, a warm, effusive woman, wanted the same warmth from her doctor. Other patients may choose a doctor whose style is quite different. For example, a patient who categorizes herself as a persuader may want to be cared for by a Marcus Welby physician; she knows what to expect from a persuader, and she wants someone who will make her feel better as well as give her top-notch care without the hype. However, it's important to recognize that doctors and patients whose styles do not match may find themselves having conflicts over communication, values, and approaches.

In addition, you may not always be able to find the doctor who exactly fits your ideal style because of a limited choice of physicians. This is especially true if you live in a small town or require a subspecialist, such as a heart or a retinal surgeon, both subspecialties in which only a few doctors are trained each year.

Just because your styles don't match perfectly is no reason to stop seeing your doctor. Both of you can work on being more flexible and accommodating. This can be done by communicating what you need from your doctor and asking what she expects from you. A doctor whose style is forceful and confident, which you may initially interpret as rude and arrogant, may later prove a source of great strength and confidence to you during difficult times. If you have a specialist who gives you the treatment you need but does not match your style, consider using your primary care physician (who hopefully matches your style) as a go-between. Exercise 2-1 at the end of the chapter will help you match your caregiver's style to your style.

<u>INSIDER'S HINT</u>

Match your personal style to your doctor's to improve your rapport and communication with your doctor.

Style Shifting As doctors mature, they may develop personality traits from categories other than their basic style. The analytic Spock may grow more empathetic, while the Scholarly Professor may learn organizational skills and social graces. A mature physician with many well-developed personality facets can better serve the patient during the shifting stages of illness. That doesn't mean you should shun the doctor right out of residency training and look for an older physician. It simply means that emotional maturity in a doctor is a plus, no matter what his or her chronological age.

In addition, your illness or condition may dictate the style or combination of styles you choose in a physician. If you are looking for hair replacement, you may not need a lot of bedside manner, and may opt for a capable persuasive charmer who runs the best hair replacement clinic in town. However, for your diabetes, a disease that can cause numerous complications and pain, you may feel more comfortable with a doctor who is a combination Marcus Welby and Spock.

Because diseases are not static, you may be best served by changing doctors as the demands of the illness change, so that the style of the physician matches the phase of the illness. For example, if you are diagnosed with cancer, initially you may select the analytic Spock to make the diagnosis and administer standard therapy. If standard therapy proves unsuccessful, you might look to the Scholarly Professor for the latest experimental treatment. If the disease progresses even in the face of the most up-to-date treatment available, you may wish to return to your primary care physician, a gentle, emotional Marcus Welby, for comfort at the end of your life. What you need changes as you change, and as your circumstances change.

CARING VERSUS CONTROLLING

No matter what your doctor's style, you deserve a doctor who cares, whether he expresses it by staying up late at night to search the medical literature to make an exact diagnosis, or through a gentle, loving touch when you most need it. A little warmth, a firm and guiding hand, and strength in times of despair and trouble can be wonderfully healing. This is medical maternalism and paternalism at its best.

But what happens when maternalism and paternalism become controlling? It is important to know the difference. Doctors need to be firm when their patients inadvertently put their lives at risk by disobeying important instructions. For example, a patient with a fungal infection that has caused an abscess in her brain informs her doctor that she has stopped taking her medication after only four weeks because she feels perfectly well. He explains that she may feel well, but her infection is still present. If she does not take the medicine for the full 52 weeks he prescribed, there's a good chance she will suffer brain damage and might even die from the infection. He explains why this is so important using his best bedside manner and clearest reasoning. But the patient insists she is well and is not willing to take the medication, because it is expensive and causes a few bothersome side-effects.

At that point, the doctor says, either take the medicine or I'll have to refer you to another physician, because I am not getting through to you. I care about you, but I am obviously not convincing you of what you need to do to maintain and improve your health. Perhaps another doctor will be more successful. Finally, the patient realizes how serious her doctor is, and she agrees to take the medication. In this situation, the doctor's firmness was the kindest behavior for the patient, though it may have seemed harsh at the time. Some circumstances, such as life-threatening illnesses, require dispensing advice and care with "tough love."

But when *care turns into control,* that is when your doctor may have crossed the line and may be doing you more harm than good. For example, a man with gout goes to his retirement party, where he drinks a bit too much alcohol and eats too much steak. That evening, his left big toe aches horribly with an attack of gout. It is perfectly appropriate for his doctor to advise strongly against drinking so much and eating red meat, because over the years this will harm the patient. But if the doctor begins to admonish the patient for the occasional, non-life threatening transgression, this may be crossing the line.

Such inappropriate warnings can have a number of ill effects on a patient. For one thing, nobody likes to be scolded. For another, like the wife who stops listening to her nagging husband, the patient may stop listening to his doctor—even when the doctor says something of grave importance. The patient knows a single transgression is not a big deal, and so he assumes if the doctor is exaggerating this danger, perhaps he can't be trusted to tell the unvarnished truth about anything.

If you get to the point where you are afraid to speak your mind without your doctor taking it as his own personal rejection or failure, if you are being bossed around and scolded rather than advised and guided, or if you feel you are no longer in the company of Father Knows Best but rather in the presence of General Patton, then chances are you are being patronized or controlled.

BEWARE IF YOU ARE TREATED IN A CONDESCENDING MANNER RATHER THAN AS AN EQUAL PARTNER IN YOUR CARE. When you become a passive player in your own medical care, you can imperil your health. All doctors can make mistakes—medicine is an art, after all. But the doctor who wants to control his patients may be especially prone to errors in judgment.

DOES YOUR DOCTOR MEET THE FOUR C'S TEST?

An important test for determining whether or not your doctor can meet your needs is determining if he manifests the four C's of medicine. In other words, is he:

Comfortable—Does he seem trustworthy and emotionally involved in your care?

Competent—Is she medically capable and up on the latest medical research?

Confident—Is he self-assured and do you feel stronger when you're around him ?

Caring—Does she listen and act with empathy?

Exercise 2-2 will help you determine how many of these characteristics your doctor displays. Ideally, he or she would embody all four characteristics. Though many care givers have some elements of each characteristic, few have them all.

How Does the Office Staff Rate?

Office staff can be viewed as an extension of the doctor's personality. Your opinion of the staff will most likely influence your opinion of the doctor. Ask yourself if you thought the office staff was friendly, efficient, and helpful. Can the receptionist answer your simple questions? Did the nurse or medical assistant act like a drill sergeant or a supportive assistant? Did the staff behave as if it was a bother to see you, or did they make you feel comfortable and ease your anxiety?

Sometimes conflicts with the staff will be enough to make you want to change doctors. If your assessment of the doctor's staff is negative but you like the doctor, then it is worth calling the doctor or writing a letter, explaining the problems you encountered with the staff. Most of the time, these letters are discussed at staff meetings and attempts are made to improve the staff's interaction with the patients. Doctors and staff may need a reminder that a patient is also a customer who could be shopping elsewhere. Doctors will try to improve the office atmosphere so the patient (customer) wants to return.

Would You Let Him Treat Your Pet?

If you are still unsure as to whether you should return to this doctor, then ask yourself one simple question: Would you let him treat your beloved pet?

- If the answer is no, then get out of there.
- If the answer is yes, then it is probably okay to continue seeing this doctor.

The most basic question is, do you trust your doctor? A lot of trust is based on respect. Likewise, respect is based on knowledge, communication, and personality. If the doctor's style fits your needs, if she communicates well with you in a way that satisfies your needs, and if you feel that she is competent and she wants to help you, then you will most likely trust her and follow her guidance and instructions.

Undesirable Doctor or Undesirable Patient?

Undesirable behavior by doctor or by patient? Sometimes it's hard to know who is to blame for poor communication. Usually, both parties must share it. So if your analysis of the doctor up to this point has resulted in a less than glowing review, you need to ask yourself: Does he have poor doctor skills or am I behaving poorly as a patient?

Doctors are professionals and should be able to ignore aspects of a person's behavior that they don't particularly like, at least in theory. In an ideal situation, a patient's behavior towards the doctor should not affect his ability to evaluate and treat the problem. But this does not always happen in the real world. If a patient spends the first half hour of his visit complaining about all of the other doctors he has seen for this problem, the physician may respond by being guarded and short with the patient. He may ask himself, "Could all of those doctors be so bad and terribly wrong?" He'll most likely think, "Probably not," and he will assume that the patient is negative and unrealistic. Not surprisingly, the doctor may decide that he doesn't want to take care of the patient, either.

ARE YOU MR. ICE?

What is poor patient behavior? Just as there are undesirable doctors there are undesirable patients. Patients who show no courtesy to staff, doctor, or other patients; patients who are late more often than not or who fail to show up for appointments at all; patients who lie or are deceitful; and patients who threaten legal action in order to manipulate the system are generally considered bad patients. For example, Mr. Ice, who is suffering from some weakness and numbness in his arm, comes in to the radiology clinic for an MRI. He refuses to cooperate with the experienced technologist, who has been appropriate and polite. Realizing that the patient is angry, the technologist asks the patient if he would like to speak to the doctor in charge.

When Mr. Ice meets the doctor, the first words out of his mouth are not hello but rather a tirade about how rude and incompetent everyone has been. He announces that he is planning to sue his surgeon, and if his scan is not performed perfectly and at the cost he expects, he will also sue the radiologist and refuse to pay the bill. The doctor recognizes that the patient is fearful, and asks him what he expects from the MRI. Mr. Ice replies that he will let the doctors perform this one test and no others, and from that test he wants to be assured that he will receive a diagnosis of his problem—today. The doctor realizes that this cannot be done and tells the patient the MRI should be performed elsewhere. The doctor calls around and discovers that there is a specialized machine at the local university that is better suited to solving the problem. The patient begrudgingly and after much complaining agrees to go to the university.

We would all like an answer immediately, and preferably after undergoing as few tests as possible. But often, medicine can't always give us what we want. Threatening lawsuits and non-payment before undergoing a test will not inspire the doctors, technologists, nurses, or office staff to give you the best possible care. Indeed, threatening behavior is a sure way for a patient to damage rapport and alienate a doctor.

On the other hand, a patient can be polite and appropriate, yet firmly insist upon and expect good care and kind service. A patient who is resolute, yet reasonable and courteous, can sometimes be inappropriately labeled a "bad" patient. On the other hand, almost all patients (especially rude ones) think they are the ones who are being reasonable. Most caregivers try to approach a conflict with a patient with an open mind. So how can a patient know when he or she is the one who is acting inappropriately?

It sounds corny, but when in doubt, remember the golden rule: "Do unto others as you would have them do unto you." The doctor-patient relationship is a partnership built on caring, trust, respect, and communication. When situations arise in which you feel you need to look out for yourself, do not hesitate to be pro-active, vigilant, and committed to wellness. But that means that you must be pulling your share of the load to get well. The doctor is not going to lay on his hands and miraculously cure your hardening of the arteries with a magic pill, especially if you still insist on smoking, eating poorly, and not exercising. You need to get involved and take personal responsibility. The doctor is your partner, a knowledgeable guide and ally, but he cannot help you if you are not fully committed to helping yourself. As a general rule, if you are willing to go the extra mile for your wellness, you can ask the same from your doctor. However, if you threaten and attempt to intimidate your doctor, it will alienate her and destroy the doctor-patient relationship.

DO YOU THINK OF YOUR DOCTOR AS A MAGICAL HEALER?

In ancient cultures, doctors were referred to as healers. These healers were expected to treat the patient's emotional and physical ailments with herbal potions and incantations. The master healer provided remedies that supposedly could prolong life and return the dying from their death. Unfortunately for modern doctors, these notions have been carried into the 20th century. It has been further perpetuated by modern western technology and television caricatures of doctors bringing people back to life from the precipice of death.

As a result, patients often have unrealistic expectations that cannot be matched by flesh and blood doctors. The end result is that many patients are dissatisfied with their doctor when the cure is not painless, and the recovery is not swift and full. Such unrealistic expectations have contributed to societal dissatisfaction with doctors as well as increased malpractice litigation. Today, many patients and families of patients believe their doctors are not competent enough, when the reality is that their doctor is probably more competent than doctors have ever been at any time in history. It is important to realize that few diseases have magical cures and even fewer doctors are wizards.

Patients also tend to think that doctors should have all the answers. However, there is not always an obvious answer to your problem. Sometimes finding out the correct diagnosis and treatment is like completing a jigsaw puzzle. It takes time to put together the right pieces and complete the picture. Just because your doctor doesn't have all of the answers all of the time doesn't mean that she is stupid. **You should pay attention to how your doctor deals with not knowing the answer.** Does she admit it freely? Does she continue to look for an answer or does she just conclude that there must be nothing wrong with you? Getting the correct diagnosis and getting cured may take a long time or may never even happen. Does she seek assistance when the treatment or diagnosis are in question? The important thing is how your physician deals with uncertainty and how she treats you during this period of "not knowing." She should be honest, open, and caring to your requests for additional help, especially if you are not getting better.

WHEN YOUR DOCTOR DOES MAKE A MISTAKE

Doctors are rarely responsible for initially making the patient ill. However, in the course of attempting to treat a patient, side effects of treatment and honest misjudgments can sometimes cause the patient even greater harm than the initial disease. Effective communication is critical during such times of mistakes in order to prevent further harm to the patient.

Yet it is during these difficult situations that communication most often breaks down. This breakdown is partly a result of the drive for perfection on both the doctor's part and the patient's. The current medical legal climate, in which doctors are sometimes sued for bad outcomes that were not the result of negligence, creates a hostile environment that promotes the idea that any unexpected or "bad" outcome is malpractice for which someone must be blamed. Doctors, too, expect perfection of themselves, and this sometimes gets in the way of being able to recognize and admit a mistake, and then take steps to correct it. It requires a healthy ego to live with the consequences of a medical error that causes an injury, or even kills a patient. It can be much easier psychologically to refuse to admit an error, or to avoid confronting a patient and his family.

Unfortunately, it is human nature to make mistakes. Most of the time, your doctor will only make an occasional minor error that won't cause patients any harm. **But if your doctor does make a mistake, it is important to decide very quickly whether or not you still trust him or her.** If the doctor admits the mistake and tries hard to prevent other errors, this is a good sign and usually means you can trust your doctor. The most important thing is for a doctor to admit the mistake and correct it as soon as possible after its discovery.

This is easiest if the doctor has a good relationship with the patient. If you are able to stay focused on getting adequate care and keep blame to a minimum, we believe you will have a better chance for recovery, and for maintaining an open, constructive relationship with your doctor. But if you are adversarial, then your doctor will be less likely to admit the error, and less able to correct it. However, if you maintain good, nonaccusatory communication during this stressful time, and your doctor *still* is unable to own up to her mistake, you may no longer be able to trust her, and you should probably find another doctor.

INSIDER'S HINT
....

Good things often take time and require asking for help. Often you must ask more than once.

DID YOU GET YOUR MONEY'S WORTH?

One of the elements to your relationship with a doctor is money. Insurance may cover most or all of your charges. But these days, most individuals contribute to their health care costs through insurance premiums, co-pays, or deductibles. So it is not unreasonable for you to ask the question, "Am I getting my money's worth?"

Deciding the answer is partly personal, but it can also be objectified to some extent. Let's consider a man who has been experiencing worsening heartburn and fatigue. His physician finds he has anemia caused by a stomach ulcer. The physician prescribes one of the newer anti-ulcer medications, confident that it will be effective. But when the man picks up his medicine at the pharmacy, he has sticker shock: $150 for 30 pills! What he doesn't realize, is that this new medication is so effective in treating ulcer disease, he won't have to suffer an expensive hospitalization and blood transfusion, not to mention the economic consequences of lost work time. Thirty years ago, before the advent of these miraculous new medications, a patient with comparable symptoms may have required surgery, specifically a vagotomy (clipping of the nerves to the stomach), and/or an antrectomy (surgical remove of part of the stomach). When viewed from this perspective, $150 seems fairly reasonable, and a patient might conclude he has gotten his "money's worth." When determining the value of any treatment consider the question: What does this treatment save me with regard to pain, time, and money?

How you perceive value is also strongly tied to your pre-illness expectations and personality. Are you outcome- or process-oriented? For example, do you perceive the outcome of your illness as curable or incurable? For some patients there must be a complete cure to feel they have gotten their money's worth. For other patients if in the process the doctor cares, does his best, works hard, and communicates well, that is value even if the cure is incomplete or temporary. For most of us, value is a combination of both outcome and process.

Medical care is inevitably expensive. The cost of your doctor's care takes into account years of training and student loan debts, 24-hour on-call accessibility, malpractice insurance costs, patient care for the uninsured, as well as office expenses. Most doctors charge their patients within a narrow range of prices. But be aware, some doctors are charging prices out of line with the going rate. If the charges seem unreasonable then discuss this with your doctor and his billing staff. Perhaps a mistake has occurred. If not, then you need to think about whether he is worth it and whether you are willing to pay those extra charges. If you are not willing to pay extra, then you will have to find another doctor.

BREAKING UP ISN'T HARD TO DO

If your final assessment is that a particular patient/doctor relationship is just not right for you, then you should break-up with your doctor. You need to put your health needs first and find a doctor who meets those needs.

There are two basic ways in which you can let your doctor know that the relationship is not going to work for you.

- First, you can communicate your frustration and try to work out the differences. If unsuccessful, you can politely explain that you are unhappy with the relationship and request a referral to someone else.
- Second, you can say nothing and find yourself a new physician. You may choose to follow-up with a letter to your previous doctor explaining the reasons you left. If you chose to never communicate your dissatisfaction to the initial doctor, after a year or two your name will likely be dropped from the computer and your records placed in the inactive file in basement storage.

How you handle this break-up just depends on how comfortable you are with telling the doctor that you are leaving and why.

YOUR DOCTOR AND THE HEALING PROCESS

A good patient/doctor relationship has a strong healing power. You deserve a doctor who is competent and caring and with whom you feel confident and comfortable. When you find a doctor with whom you are happy and who satisfies your requirements, we recommend you stick with, nurture, and strengthen that relationship.

INSIDER'S HINT
There is a healing power in a healthy patient/doctor relationship.

Style Matching

This exercise can be used to identify your style and your doctor's style. First answer the questions as they apply to you. Then, if you wish, you can answer these questions as you believe they would apply to your optimal doctor.

IDENTIFYING YOUR STYLE

For each question, rate your answer from 1 to 4 (4 = most preferable; 1 = least preferable).

1. Which attribute best describes you:
____ (A) Emotional; communicate through feelings and emotions
____ (B) Analytical; communicate objectively with logic and rational thinking
____ (C) Scholarly; communicate creatively with new ideas, thoughts, and opinions
____ (D) Charismatic; communicate with charm and persuasion

2. To whom would you most trust your life? Someone who is:
____ (A) Friendly, compassionate, and caring
____ (B) Logical, organized, and principled
____ (C) Imaginative, creative, and experimental
____ (D) Persuasive, charming, and free-spirited

3. Which trait do you most admire in a doctor?
____ (A) Kindness
____ (B) Responsibility
____ (C) Creativity
____ (D) Convincing

4. Which items do you prefer to keep on your office walls?
____ (A) Pictures of family and loved ones
____ (B) Awards, honors, and diplomas
____ (C) Books, papers, or drawings of new and creative ideas
____ (D) Photos or mementos of fun trips, successful experiences, or hobbies

For each question above, add together all of the A's, then all of the B's, then all of the C's, and finally all of the D's. Record the totals for each letter category below. The letter with the highest score is your style and the doctor's style that matches you. Remember, you and your doctors may be a mixture of styles.

EXERCISE 2-1

Style Matching *(cont.)*

_____ **(A) Emotional–Marcus Welby:** This doctor functions on an emotional basis and communicates through feelings.

_____ **(B) Analytic–Mr. Spock:** This doctor functions on an analytic basis and communicates objectively through logical thoughts and opinions.

_____ **(C) Imaginative–Scholarly Professor:** This doctor functions on a scholarly and imaginative basis and communicates about the most up to date research and creative methods.

_____ **(D) Persuasive–The Persuasive Charmer:** This doctor functions by persuasion and communicates through influence and adaptation to the situation.

IDENTIFYING YOUR CURRENT PHYSICIAN'S STYLE

You can use this second part of the exercise to help clarify further your current doctor's style. (You can also answer the questions as they would apply to your optimal doctor.) For each doctor style listed below, score each trait with either a 1 if your doctor exhibits it or a 0 if he does not exhibit it. Total the scores for each style. The highest score indicates your doctor's primary style. Remember all doctors will exhibit some traits from each style, but they will have a dominant style which will influence their treatment of you.

MARCUS WELBY
_____ Compassionate approach to you
_____ Warm, friendly, and listens well
_____ Nurturing but not paternalistic or maternalistic
_____ Pictures of family on desk or walls
_____ Can become overly emotional and dramatic
_____ **Total Score**

SPOCK
_____ Takes organized analytic approach to your case
_____ Accurate and logical in communication
_____ Responsible to you and your needs
_____ Awards and diplomas fill the office
_____ Can become humorless and overly compulsive
_____ **Total Score**

Style Matching *(cont.)*

SCHOLARLY PROFESSOR
____ Creative and imaginative about your case
____ Nice enough, but no strong emotional bond
____ Appears often to be in deep thought
____ Journals and papers lying on the desk
____ Can become shy and withdrawn
____ **Total Score**

THE PERSUASIVE CHARMER
____ Resourceful and convincing in his approach
____ Demonstrative, persuasive, yet charming
____ Appears to be adaptable
____ Office reflects hobbies and interests
____ Can become aggressive and hostile
____ **Total Score**

MATCHING STYLES

You now should match the style you prefer with your doctor's style. If the style selections are different, you will need to make a decision about whether your current physician will be able to meet your needs. This exercise can also be used to help with doctor-patient communication by understanding perceived differences.

Your Style _____

Your Current Doctor's Style _____

Your Optimal Doctor's Style _____

ADDITIONAL COMMENTS

_____

_____   _____

_____

_____

_____

_____

EXERCISE 2-2

Does Your Doctor Have the 4 C's?

Write down the answer to each of the four traits

2 = yes, almost all the time; 1 = yes, sometimes; 0 = not often

COMFORTABLE

____ Does your doctor help you to feel safe and secure?

____ Do you have good gut feelings about him as a person

____ Do you have good gut feelings about him as a doctor?

____ Do you trust him?

____ Do you view him as an ally?

____ **Total**

COMPETENT

____ Does your doctor have the skill and ability to properly diagnose you?

____ Does she behave in a professional manner?

____ Do you respect her expertise?

____ Did she provide you with a good treatment plan?

____ Does she follow through with your treatment and adjust it as needed?

____ **Total**

CONFIDENT

____ Does your doctor exhibit self-assuredness without being arrogant?

____ Does he appear comfortable with his style, skills, and abilities?

____ Does she appear comfortable answering your questions?

____ If she doesn't know an answer, can she admit to it and tell you she will need help from others?

____ Does she empower you?

____ **Total**

EXERCISE 2-2

Does Your Doctor Have the 4 C's? *(cont.)*

CARING

_____ Does your doctor listen to you?

_____ Does she empathize with you?

_____ Can she communicate to you in an understanding and compassionate manner?

_____ Does she take into consideration your feelings and thoughts?

_____ Does she understand your moral, ethical, and religious dilemmas?

_____ **Total**

If the totals for each group are: **7 to 10 = yes**, check the applicable category below; **4 to 6 = maybe**, check the applicable category below; **0 to 3 = no**, do not check the applicable category below.

_____ Comfortable   _____ Confident

_____ Competent   _____ Caring

4 C's: Excellent match   2 C's: Fair match

3 C's: Good match   1 C: Poor match

3 to 4 = Excellent Match. If your doctor has all four of these characteristics, that is great. You have probably found the right doctor for you.

2 to 3 = Good Match. If he has three of the characteristics, that is good. You just need to make sure that the missing characteristic is not a crucial one to you.

1 to 2 = Fair Match. If your doctor has only two characteristics, then you might want to think about changing doctors. If he has the two characteristics you consider to be the most important, you may want to try to make the relationship work.

0 to 1 = Poor Match. If your doctor has only one characteristic, you will probably be served better by another doctor.

Chapter 3

Is It Time for a Second Opinion?

Cindy Horn knew something was wrong, but what? For weeks she had been suffering with muscle pain all over, poor sleep, fatigue, and numerous other problems. Finally, a diagnosis was made. Cindy's rheumatologist told her she had fibromyalgia, a chronic, benign disorder. Cindy had never heard of fibromyalgia before, but she was relieved her symptoms had a name and that it wasn't a fatal disease.

When Cindy got home, she immediately sat down and read all of the fibromyalgia literature her doctor had given her. Beginning that day, she started to make some of the recommended lifestyle modifications. She began eating better and started a daily exercise and stretch routine. After about a month, Cindy did notice some improvement, but she still did not feel like her old self. A single question nagged her, "What if the doctor's assessment is wrong?" For her own peace of mind, she decided to see another rheumatologist after talking with her primary care doctor.

The second rheumatologist asked Cindy many of the same questions she had been asked before. In fact, the exams were almost identical. However, the second rheumatologist appeared to focus on something the other doctor had not—Cindy's sleep patterns. After many questions, the second rheumatologist verified that Cindy did indeed have fibromyalgia. However, for her, the fibromyalgia was aggravated by a sleep disorder called "nocturnal myoclonus," which results in fibromyalgia in many but not all patients. It turned out that Cindy was having abnormal muscular contractions at night that interfered with her sleep, causing the fatigue and musculoskeletal pain of fibromyalgia pain. A new treatment plan was prescribed, and Cindy's search for a second opinion paid off with improved health.

TWO HEADS CAN BE BETTER THAN ONE

A second opinion is just that, an opinion. Medicine is not a precise science. Instead, it is more of a skill and an art that often involves some trial and error. There are times when it is important to seek a second opinion to verify for yourself that your diagnosis or treatment plan is correct. The second opinion can, in fact, save your life if the original diagnosis is wrong. However, more often than not, the second opinion simply provides you with:

- Confidence in your original diagnosis and treatment
- Confidence in your original physician
- Additional information concerning your disease and care

WHY A SECOND OPINION?

There are a variety of reasons for seeking a second opinion.

YOU ARE NOT RESPONDING TO TREATMENT. If you have been under your doctor's care for some time and your symptoms have not responded to treatment as expected, then it might be time for a second opinion. For example, maybe you're feeling tired, weak, and depressed. Your doctor has given you medication for the depression, and you do feel a bit better, but the fatigue persists. A second opinion diagnoses a low thyroid condition. You receive thyroid hormone replacement treatment and all of your symptoms resolve.

YOU LACK CONFIDENCE IN YOUR PHYSICIAN. Confidence can be based on many factors other than your doctor's competence. In fact, your doctor might be quite competent and medically knowledgeable, but if you perceive your doctor isn't very sure of herself or the diagnosis, you might want a second opinion. Perhaps you just don't like your doctor or don't share the same communication style. As a result, you find yourself questioning her judgment, diagnosis, and treatment plan. If you reach this point, a second opinion is recommended. If the diagnosis and treatment are confirmed, your confidence in your doctor may get a boost. Or, you might find the second doctor more to your liking and change physicians.

YOU NEED REASSURANCE ABOUT TREATMENT OPTIONS. If you are facing a significant surgery or risky procedure, a second opinion may reassure you that there is not a better, less invasive, or safer option. Some doctors recommend only traditional treatments, but if you would like to explore the possibility of a non-traditional approach, then a second opinion might be in order. The same is true if you think your doctor is focusing too much on a non-traditional or experimental treatment and you would feel more comfortable with a traditional approach. You owe yourself a second opinion to convince yourself that a potentially better treatment has not been overlooked.

YOUR PHYSICIAN ASKS YOU TO GET A SECOND OPINION. Doctors are pretty astute. If they're not sure of a diagnosis, not getting the results they expect, or sense you do not have confidence in them or their treatment plan, they'll usually send you to another doctor they respect, who is equally or more knowledgeable about the health issue. This second doctor may know of some care that was not considered. Sometimes it takes a fresh perspective from another physician to find the "forest through the trees."

YOUR INSURANCE COMPANY REQUIRES IT. Many insurance plans require a second opinion for elective surgeries. Elective surgeries are those that are scheduled at your convenience and are not performed immediately, as in the case of emergencies. There also might be other reasons why an insurance company requires a second opinion. To determine when you need a second opinion, review your insurance company's explanation of benefits booklet.

MEDICO-LEGAL OPINIONS. Legal or administrative issues may be another reason to see another doctor. Medico-legal opinions are different from true second opinions because they are not for the purpose of recommending treatment. Rather, they are used to confirm a diagnosis or to help establish causation for medico-legal purposes. For example, say you are in an auto accident. Most likely your own physician would examine and treat your injuries. To satisfy insurance or court requirements, though, a second opinion from another doctor may be required, especially if a lawsuit is involved.

DOCTOR SHOPPING. Finally, some people seek a second opinion because they disagree with a certain diagnosis or treatment. They go "doctor shopping," looking for a doctor that will tell them what they want to hear. Third, fourth, and fifth opinions usually serve little purpose other than to rack up expenses and muddle care. The right words can make you feel emotionally better, but they don't necessarily make you feel physically better.

ASKING FOR A SECOND OPINION

We recommend that you ask your current doctor for a referral for a second opinion. Resist feeling awkward or uncomfortable doing this, it is perfectly appropriate. If your doctor acts insulted and overly defensive, he may be putting his ego ahead of your well being, and he might not be the best doctor for you. Many doctors will recommend another doctor or two when asked for a referral. This is helpful because there is an excellent chance that your first doctor will listen to and respect that second opinion, even if it differs from hers. You shouldn't worry that the referring doctor will just tell the second opinion doctor what to say and what to recommend. This is rare. Physicians do abide by the Hippocratic code of ethics to "do no harm" to the patient. If the second opinion truly differs from the first, you should be told.

At the least, you should tell your doctor that you are going for a second opinion. Even if you don't say a thing, he will almost certainly know when he is asked to send your medical records to another office. If you prefer that your doctor not know, follow the guidelines in Chapter 6, and be prepared to provide the second doctor with copies of your medical records.

WHAT ABOUT THE EXPERTS?

When people think about second opinions they often picture seeing the mythical "best" specialist in the country. Many times they seek out their friend's "guru" or the so-called expert who hawks miracle cures on TV. This certainly is an option, but it may not be necessary or wise. Self-promoted cures may prove expensive if not dangerous to your well being.

Experts exist at all levels—local, state, and national. An excellent choice for specialty care is a local specialty center that focuses on specific diseases and treatments, such as a women's health clinic or cancer center. Medical centers and university-based teaching hospitals will usually satisfy a broad range of patient needs, particularly for rare and esoteric diseases requiring unusual or experimental treatments.

Many community physicians have affiliations with universities or conduct state-of-the-art medical research but have chosen the private sector. Ask your community specialty center about its university or academic affiliations. The gap between the university physician and the community physician has narrowed in recent years, especially in larger cities, as more and more former university professors seek private medical practices. Furthermore, for many routine procedures, a patient may be better treated by a community doctor who performs the procedure hundreds of times than at a university where the treatment in performed, at least in part, by providers still in training.

If the regional university hospital is stumped, you might want to go to a nationally-known institution. Medical meccas such as the Mayo and Cleveland clinics and the National Institutes of Health attract and employ top experts in many areas of medicine. In fact, doctors at these centers are often super-specialized. They concentrate their practice and research in well-defined specialized areas of medicine. In the case of rare diseases, these doctors may see more of a particular disease in a year than your doctor sees in a lifetime. These national meccas also might be the place to go if you are having trouble getting a definitive diagnosis or if standard therapy is failing.

At medical meccas, you are examined by experts in several disciplines who coordinate the work-up and reach a consensus decision. This approach may provide you with "The Answer" if one has not been forthcoming. These physicians may also be developing experimental therapies not available to community physicians. For more information on how to contact these meccas, see page 88.

WHO PAYS FOR A SECOND OPINION?

Who pays for a second opinion depends on your insurance coverage or lack thereof. If the opinion is required by the insurance company prior to an elective surgery, it will be covered. Otherwise, it usually is covered as is any other consultation in accordance with your insurance policy. It should be noted that some insurance policies and managed care programs require prior authorization or a referral from your primary physician in order for you to be covered. We recommend you call your insurance company or primary physician to find this out before seeking the second opinion.

If you believe you need a second opinion and your insurance company doesn't, then you will have to pay for it yourself. If your second opinion proves to be at odds with your initial diagnosis, then you might try going back to your insurance company and prove to them that the second opinion was justified. With some persistence, you might be able to convince them to cover the second opinion.

To avoid problems, make sure you get the appropriate prior authorization and referral documents before getting a second opinion.

DOES A SECOND OPINION MEAN A REPEAT OF TESTS?

Keeping good personal medical records may help to keep repeat diagnostic testing to a minimum. (See Chapter 8 for information on preparing your medical history.) But if it's been a while since your last lab work, repeat testing may be ordered to evaluate changes.

Some tests are repeated in order to follow the course and progress of a disease and its care. Tests that were negative before may now be positive and vice versa. Additionally, test results can vary between laboratories, so your doctor may only feel comfortable with a lab or personnel she trusts. For example, a biopsy reading or an MRI evaluation require a high degree of human judgment and experience. A decision for surgery may need to be based on a new test or x-ray. Finally, you need to remember that all tests need to be interpreted in conjunction with the clinical exam, which may be different in a second opinion visit.

BECAUSE THE EXPERT SAYS IT'S SO, DOESN'T MAKE IT SO

Two heads are usually, but not always, better than one. A second opinion may not always be correct. Here again, you need to remember that medicine is more art than science. It could be that the second doctor is making the error in judgment. If this seems like it could be frustrating or frightening, you're right, it is.

Several possible outcomes can occur when you seek a second opinion.

- The second opinion can agree with your present diagnosis and treatment.
- The second opinion can agree with some but not all of the elements of your present diagnosis and treatment.
- The second opinion can conflict with your present diagnosis and treatment.

So what should you do if the second opinion differs from or conflicts with the original diagnosis or treatment? Who is right? Do you hire yet another doctor for a tie-breaker?

There is no clear answer. You must decide which course to follow using your knowledge of the illness and confidence in the doctor. If the differences are minor, your primary doctor can review the new information and perhaps adjust the diagnosis and treatment as is appropriate. If the opinions do not agree or lead to a common approach, we recommend that you ask the two doctors to discuss the case and devise a common plan of action. If the differences are great, you may be forced to decide between the two doctors or seek a third tie-breaking opinion. Exercise 3-1 will help you sort out this information.

EXERCISE 3-1

Second Opinion
FIRST OPINION
Physician's Name: _____

Diagnosis: _____

Treatment Plan: _____

SECOND OPINION
Physician's Name: _____

Diagnosis: _____

Treatment Plan: _____

CHOOSING YOUR COURSE
Are the diagnoses the same or different? _____

If they are different, how are they different?_____
_____

Which diagnosis do you believe and trust?_____

Why do you believe and trust this diagnosis?_____
_____

Are the treatment plans the same or different?_____

If they are different, how are they different?_____
_____

Which treatment plan do you think you will follow and why?_____
_____

What does your own research tell you regarding your condition
and how does it compare to the two different opinions? _____
_____

Is there an alternative treatment the doctor will not administer
which you would like to try? Why won't the doctor give you the
treatment? _____
_____

What is your gut reaction to the two different doctors? _____
_____

Are you confident with their expertise and skills? _____

Chapter 4

The Internet

Jim's mother-in-law, Beth, was diagnosed with amyloidosis at age 67. Amyloidosis is a rare disease that kills most people within two months to two years of onset. Beth's doctor had never treated a patient with amyloidosis during his 24 years of practice and knew little about the disease or treatments.

Out of frustration, Jim decided to learn everything he could to help Beth. In years past, Jim would have gone to the library and searched through the stacks of literature to find applicable articles. But that was before the Information Age.

Jim went first to the Internet. Within days, he learned what it meant to have amyloidosis, and soon had the names and telephone numbers of the doctors who were world experts on the disease. Excited by this information, Jim called one of the experts in Canada. That doctor was able to refer him to an American expert in Boston.

At the same time that Jim was surfing the Internet for medical facts, he was also gathering personal opinions and testimony. Jim had put out a global call for help by e-mail via a newsgroup's web site. To his delight, a newsgroup user, Tom, e-mailed hopeful news. Tom indicated that before his treatment, he had been restricted to a sedentary life with little hope of survival. But now two years later, after treatment for amyloidosis of the heart, he was probably cured and felt healthy enough to referee his son's soccer game. Even better, Tom's treatment was administered by the same Boston physician recommended by the Canadian expert.

With this glimmer of hope, Jim called the Boston physician. The doctor explained the risks and benefits of the treatment. It cured about 20 percent of all patients, but it was both experimental and dangerous. Still, if begun in the early stages of the disease, the new treatment did offer some hope where previously none had existed before.

Jim took this new found information to his mother-in-law, Beth. She was very grateful but felt she was too old to undergo such radical therapy. Instead, Beth chose to let nature take its course and she died within six months.

Jim thought Beth's death signaled the end of any involvement with amyloidosis. That is, until one day while reviewing the amyloidosis newsgroup messages out of curiosity he ran across an electronic cry for help. Alice, a 42-year-old mother of young children, had just been diagnosed with amyloidosis of the heart and was given little hope for survival past a year. Her husband Peter had posted the "electronic message in a bottle" asking for help. Jim immediately responded, and suggested they contact the physician in Boston. The woman and her family now were aware of the possibility of a cure, something they might not have known about without the Internet.

HEALTH CARE ALONG THE ELECTRONIC SUPERHIGHWAY

The Internet has opened up a whole new realm of health care information for patients and doctors alike. People on opposite sides of the globe, who otherwise would never meet, are now communicating electronically, exchanging information and opinions.

Information is vital. It is the life-blood of modern medicine. It can mean the difference between getting well or staying ill. It is imperative that if you want to get well and stay well, you not only educate yourself but also help educate your doctor about your illness.

With the Internet, no longer must patients depend on one doctor's knowledge or opinion. The Internet allows patients to become better informed about their illnesses. It gives them the courage to ask questions about their diagnosis and treatment and seek care elsewhere, if they feel it is warranted.

The Internet is also a global message center. If illness isolates, then the Internet is a means for ending that isolation. One of the great powers of the Internet is that it allows unrelated individuals to exchange experiences and information directly. It provides the means for patients—who often feel like shipwrecked victims—to find, share, and empower each other through communication. The Internet is already becoming an extended cyber-family giving encouragement and solace to individuals with common illnesses.

A brief note of caution: The quality of information on the Internet can vary greatly. Someone's opinion might be comforting but not necessarily medically valid.

Many books and other resources are available if you are unfamiliar with the technical aspects of accessing the Internet. There are also a number of books that cover on-line health information, including *Health Online* by Tom Ferguson, *Health & Medicine on the Internet* edited by James B. Davis, and *Mosby's Medical Surfari*. In this book, however, we will focus on finding and using the best sources of health information.

WHAT INFORMATION IS AVAILABLE?
WHERE SHOULD I LOOK?

Use any of the Internet's search engines and you'll find information on everything from AIDS to zymogenesis. Of course, it won't all be reliable. In fact, the freedom of expression the Internet provides may also be its greatest weakness. Individuals or groups can say almost anything they desire, so there is no guarantee that the information is correct or accurate. It is therefore best to consider the source of the information.

The most reliable sources of information come from:
- Libraries and their collective databases, such as MEDLINE.
- Universities, such as the University of Washington.
- Professional medical associations, such as the American Medical Association.
- National support organizations, such as the American Cancer Society.
- Government departments and agencies, such as the Centers for Disease Control.

These are the best places to look to first for reliable and useful information.

In general, newsgroups are less reliable sources of medical information. Still, they can be helpful, especially for connecting with others that may be facing the same health problem as you. A newsgroup functions as a community bulletin board at a local grocery or the town hall. It facilitates the exchange of information and opinions about any topic, medical or otherwise. You can tack up what you want, when you want.

The reliability of the newsgroups is determined by the reliability of the moderator overseeing the bulletin board. However, most newsgroups are not moderated. The end result often is the posting of unreliable and suspect information. The same goes for mailing lists, chat rooms, and some commercial or for-profit web sites, especially those that charge fees for medical information or sell treatment programs or miracle drugs. You must beware of the quacks and hucksters who are out to make a buck by preying on people looking for medical help.

A web site called Deja News (http://dejanews.com) has been created to search only for newsgroups. Mailing lists, also called Listservs, are similar to newsgroups. However, instead of getting information posted to a bulletin board, the information is e-mailed to a subscriber's account. To find a mailing list try Liszt Select (http://www.liszt.com).

Not only should you be leery of the individual selling a medical cure you also need to watch out for people who are posting false and damaging information. Anyone with access to a computer can start their own home page and espouse their own science and opinions. If a web page is written by a single, unknown individual, then you should exercise caution when using the information. A web site that is developed by a team or an organization, especially one that is well-known and well-regarded, is going to be a more reliable and trustworthy source of information. If you do come across information from a single source that sounds promising, then we suggest that you do another search around that piece of information. More information certainly can't hurt, and hopefully it will guide you to a good health decision.

Exercise 4-1 will help you to get started on your search using the Internet.

WELL-RESPECTED HEALTH-RELATED WEB SITES

AMERICAN CANCER SOCIETY http://www.cancer.org—Provides information and news about cancer and treatments.

AMERICAN MEDICAL ASSOCIATION http://www.ama-assn.org—Provides a searchable database and links to other sites.

CENTERS FOR DISEASE CONTROL http://www.cdc.gov

FOOD AND DRUG ADMINISTRATION http://www.fda.gov—Provides notices of drug and medical device approvals.

HEALTH ATOZ http://www.healthatoz.com—A very good general starting point for medical information. Good for both medical search novices and experts who want to learn more about specific diseases.

HEALTHFINDER http://www.healthfinder.gov—Provides access to federal, state, nonprofit and other sites and acts as an organizer. Its domain is the U.S. Department of Health and Human Services.

KIDSHEALTH http://www.kidshealth.org—Well organized information about children.

MAYO'S HEALTH OASIS http://www.mayo.ivi.com

MEDICONSULT http://www.mediconsult.com—A moderated site that provides information from government and medical sources.

MEDLINE http://www.nlm.nih.gov—The National Library of Medicine provides this free service providing extensive and current expert medical information and publications.

MEDSCAPE http://www.medscape.com—Provides a searchable database of credible sources.

NATIONAL LIBRARY OF MEDICINE http://www.nlm.nih.gov—Produces the electronic bibliography called Medline, which can be accessed from many sites for no charge.

NEW ENGLAND JOURNAL OF MEDICINE http://www.nejm.org—Provides access to journal articles.

OBGYN.NET http://www.obgyn.net—Doctor-reviewed site that provides ob/gyn information.

ONCOLINK http://www.oncolink.com—An excellent source of information about cancer and cancer related treatments.

PSYCH CENTRAL http://www.grohol.com—Information on mental health issues.

US PHARMACOPOEIA http://www.housecall.com—Provides information from the nation's standard drug reference.

How to Use Information from the Internet

It's becoming more and more common for people to see their doctors armed with pages upon pages of information gleaned from the Internet.

The thought of giving a doctor advice or questioning his knowledge or decisions creates discomfort for many people, especially those who grew up in households where a doctor's word was not challenged. Many individuals believe a doctor is an expert whose authority is not to be questioned or judged. But times are changing, and now more than ever it is important for patients to carefully examine the advice and decisions of their doctors. The trick is, how can you assert your rights and express your opinion comfortably, yet avoid insulting and bruising a doctor's ego?

Start by realizing that accurate information is a gift that both you and your doctor should use to improve your health and care.

FIRST, IT MAY BE MORE PRODUCTIVE TO VIEW YOUR DOCTOR AS A KNOWLEDGEABLE TEACHER WHOSE KNOWLEDGE IS EXTENSIVE BUT CONSTANTLY REQUIRING UPDATING, instead of approaching doctors as omniscient. In general, teachers and doctors enjoy learning. Patients who can teach their doctors factual information that is well researched and accurate will usually be appreciated. Those who peddle misinformation and unsubstantiated or unverifiable reports will be viewed poorly and may not be taken seriously in the future. Therefore, it is vitally important that you be prepared with medical facts, not tabloid or Internet trash.

SECOND, IT IS VALUABLE TO RECOGNIZE THAT DOCTORS MAKE MISTAKES. Most of these mistakes are correctable. System errors occur frequently because of the inherent complexity and inefficiency of the health care delivery system. A well-informed patient who asks judicious questions serves as a kind of quality control for doctors. Knee jerk obedience rather than thinking leads to errors that may prove dangerous to your health. It is disconcerting, to say the least, that 10 percent of hospital cardiac arrests are attributable to medication errors and that daily medication error rates in hospitals of have been documented to be as high as 12 percent.

FINALLY, MORE AND MORE CONFLICTS OF INTEREST ARE ARISING WHICH DEMAND THAT PATIENTS PROACTIVELY DEFEND THEIR HEALTH CARE RIGHTS. Many doctors currently are being asked to serve two masters, their patient and an insurance company or health organization that limits the care a doctor can provide (see Chapter 15). This means that doctors may not always have only the patient's interest in mind.

INFORMATION SHARING

After you have done your homework and gathered accurate information, it's time to present your doctor with your findings. Your doctor should welcome the information you present so long as it represents high quality research and is presented respectfully and in a spirit of cooperation. Names and phone numbers of experts will enhance your presentation and make your comments more palatable and credible. Remember, you are simply sharing information. Let your doctor review the information. Then listen to her response:

A doctor who is secure in her knowledge and treatment will appreciate the effort. She may or may not agree with the information or judgment of others, but she should be able to explain why she believes her medical opinion is the correct one.

If her medical position sounds plausible and you accept her explanations, then you are more likely to feel a sense of control and partnership in future decisions. After your research is completed you may discover that your doctor's care is superb and in accord with the best medical and Internet minds. This can create confidence in your doctors and their treatment plan.

If you cannot accept his explanation or think you require care other than what is prescribed, then you may need to seek a second opinion or change doctors (see Chapter 3). This may also be necessary if your doctor will not explain himself or is threatened by your research.

As you look to the Internet and other sources for medical information, keep in mind that a little knowledge can be dangerous. Isolated facts and anecdotal stories need to be put into their proper prospective. They may be misleading and not represent the full picture. Reports of new procedures and medications frequently are greeted with unbridled excitement, only later to be proven less effective than the initial hype. We recommend that for all new information you first scrutinize the facts carefully and then attempt to understood how they apply to your situation, before you incorporate the new concepts into the tapestry of your medical care.

INSIDER'S HINT

When you present Internet information to your doctor in a thoughtful and organized manner, it can educate your doctor and positively influence your care.

EXERCISE 4-1

The Internet

It is beyond the scope of this book to instruct you in the use of the Internet; however, we do have some helpful hints.

Getting Started It is actually fairly easy to browse the Internet. The on-line commercial services such as Microsoft Network, America Online, Compuserve, and Prodigy provide Internet access and connections (links) that help guide you through the web. Once on-line, use one of the search engines, such as Lycos (http//:www.lycos.com) or Yahoo (http//:www. yahoo.com) to search the desired web site.

To access a web site, type in the web address. For example the web site address for the website health AtoZ is http//:www.healthatoz. com. Once you have been connected to the web site follow the prompts and instructions provided. Below is a sample subject search.

Subject Search Here is an example of how to access a web site and search for medical information. Using Medline, you can gather facts about laser surgery for diabetic induced retinopathy, an eye disorder. Our example utilizes healthatoz.com, a user friendly medical web site.

In the Address Box: Type www.healthatoz.com   Hit <return>

Click On *Medline*.

In the Box marked *for*, type the words:

> *diabetes* and *eye* and *laser*
> (Put a space and the word *and* after each key word)

Click on the number of years to be included in the search.

Click on *Search*.

Click on the reference you desire to review.

For additional instructions, click on search tips.

You can use these instructions as a template for your personalized search by substituting your condition and the information needed for the words in italics. If you have prostate cancer and want to find out about radiation treatment with radioactive seeds, then make the following substitutions:

substitute *cancer* for *diabetes*
substitute *prostate* for *eye*
substitute *radiation* and *seeds* for *laser*

Chapter 5

Am I Really Sick?

T.J. became short of breath after climbing a few flights of stairs. He knew he wasn't the poster boy for physical fitness. After all, he was a 46-year-old stressed out, overweight, hypertensive computer programmer whose most vigorous exercise for 10 years had been "surfing the Internet." Despite all this, he wasn't really concerned about his health because he had undergone a complete physical exam three years earlier, which included a stress test of the heart that had come back as "normal."

Nevertheless, T.J. vowed to take better care of himself by cutting down on his smoking, improving his diet, and beginning a regular exercise program. He chose to start his new and healthier lifestyle with jogging because he had enjoyed it in college. One day, after about 15 minutes of jogging, he began to experience a burning pressure in his chest. He stopped, and within a few minutes the pressure subsided. He decided to continue his run, attributing his symptoms to the heart burn he had felt on and off for six months.

One week later, T.J. collapsed while jogging. He was admitted to the hospital with a mild heart attack. As he lay in the coronary care unit, T.J. reflected on the last decade and wondered how he had gone from a state of health to one of illness.

Should you just take two aspirin and go to bed, or will you die before morning? No doubt there have been times in your life when you felt practically near death. But then you took some aspirin, got bedrest, and felt much better in the morning. It can be difficult deciding if you are sick; how sick you really are; and whether you need to pick up the telephone and call your doctor. This chapter is designed to help you answer those questions.

So, Am I Sick?

Symptoms are the bodies warning signals. Any change from what you normally experience could be considered a potential symptom. The trouble is, a potential symptom of what? Are these changes the acceptable normal variations of daily living or are they the first stages of an illness. Symptoms are not always easy to understand.

Even if you are a genius, you may not understand your symptoms. Take the case of Jim Henson, Kermit and Miss Piggy's "father," who died May 15th, 1990.

Several days before he died, Jim Henson developed a sore throat. A fever and a cough followed. Like many people, he did not run to the doctor. A sore throat and cough usually pass, and just require extra fluids and rest. But then he became short of breath and more ill. By the time he went to the hospital he had developed severe pneumonia. Six antibiotics were started, but they take up to 48 hours to help. Jim Henson didn't have 48 hours. Twenty hours after arriving at the hospital, and four days after first feeling a sore throat, Jim Henson went into shock and died.

Retelling Jim Henson's story isn't meant to frighten you. But there are times when a strep throat is caused by a bacteria called Group A Streptococcus, which acts in an aggressive fashion, multiplies rapidly, and triggers a huge immune response. But how can you know the difference between a simple cold or potentially fatal infection? How could Jim Henson have known?

Having intelligence and resources alone are not enough. You must develop a means of evaluating your state of health and your need for routine or emergency care. Were there signs that could have alerted Jim Henson to his danger? Maybe, maybe not. His illness was easy to detect, but its seriousness was difficult to assess in the first 48 hours.

At the other extreme, an illness that comes on slowly can sometimes be difficult to detect. Symptoms may progress insidiously and either go undetected or be "explained away" with excuses like not getting enough sleep, being stressed, or just getting old. It is when a slowly progressive illness begins to interfere with normal life either by creating pain or interfering with bodily functions that it is usually detected and must be heeded.

INSIDER'S HINT

Symptoms are the bodies warning signals. Listen to their message.

As you evaluate any changes (symptoms) in your body, consider their severity by noticing:
- The level of pain and suffering
- The level of interference with normal bodily functions (dysfunction)
- How long the pain and the dysfunction have lasted

The greater any one of these factors, the more abnormal and potentially dangerous the symptoms and the more likely it is that you are sick.

ASSESSING YOUR HEALTH AND ILLNESS

Health can be approached from both an objective and subjective perspective. An accurate assessment of your wellness requires that both perspectives be adequately evaluated. The objective perspective deals more with measurable observable findings such as temperature, blood pressure, lab tests, and x-rays. The subjective perspective deals more with feelings, intuition, concerns, and symptoms such as pain which are not easily measured. In order to determine if you are sick and how sick you are, you need to assess both the objective data and your subjective awareness of what is normal for you.

1. ARE THESE SYMPTOMS NORMAL OR ABNORMAL?

This is the pivotal question in all of medicine. "Normal" is a concept that is difficult to define. Determining when a condition is normal and when it is abnormal may sound simple, but it can be one of the most difficult tasks in medicine for both doctors and patients.

THE PHYSICIAN'S (MEDICAL) PERSPECTIVE OF NORMAL: NORMAL OBJECTIVE TESTING = HEALTHY In general, doctors think that if your physical exam and measurable laboratory tests are normal, then you should be normal. The doctor's perspective of normal is based on comparing what you are experiencing to what everyone around you is experiencing. It is the world of physical exams and laboratory test results. Normal values and results vary between individuals, populations, circumstances, and time of life. For example, gray hair at age 20 is abnormal whereas at age 60, it is normal. Doctors are taught to evaluate people with respect to "normal" and "abnormal physical findings," "lab values," and diagnostic tests. The results of your testing are then compared to that of similar findings in a large group of age, sex, and race matched individuals.

It is important to remember that all medical tests are imperfect and can produce false positive results (says you are sick when you are not sick) and false negative results (says you are well when you are not well). A vigilant awareness that objective testing is imperfect coupled with an awareness that a disease can be present but undetectable sometimes limits the value of the objective perspective.

THE PATIENT'S PERSPECTIVE OF NORMAL: FEELING HEALTHY = NORMAL In general, patients think that if they feel healthy then everything must be normal. However, as you know, it is possible to feel well yet still have disease developing and endangering a person's welfare (heart disease). We can define normal or healthy as a condition in which the body can be exposed to stress and yet still function in a healthy and relatively pain-free manner. Wellness can be thought of like a rubber band. If you are healthy your body possesses a resiliency and an ability to adjust to different stresses. If your body encounters enough stress or illness it may fail to return to its youthful or normal resiliency. Each person differs in their ability to fight disease. Exercise 5-1 will help you determine what is "normal" for you.

If the symptoms are normal for your current state of health then you probably either are not sick or will likely not seek a doctor for assistance. But if the symptoms are abnormal than you should ask the next question.

2. HOW ABNORMAL ARE THESE SYMPTOMS?
HOW CONCERNED SHOULD I BE?

These two questions are linked together. They combine the objective and subjective perspective of your condition. Level of concern is the mind's call to action. Concern is a subjective perspective. This is the "gut feeling" as to how well or ill a person believes he or she is.

LEVELS OF CONCERN

- Minimal to No Concern/Healthy— At this level, you feel healthy and vigorous and there are few if any symptoms present.

- Moderate Concern—At this level of concern, symptoms may be mild, moderate, or severe. The symptoms generate a level of moderate concern and worry that something is wrong and needs to be corrected. Even so, no real sense of danger exists at this time.
- Substantial Concern/Danger—At this level, the symptoms have become severe enough to trigger a sense of "real" danger. You realize that some underlying disease may exist and be serious enough that it might even result in permanent disabling or damaging effects to your body or lifestyle.

MINIMAL TO NO CONCERN/HEALTHY The level of Minimal to No Concern/ Healthy includes that elusive, ideal state of perfect health in which every aspect of our body is functioning flawlessly. It is often said that the healthy person just has not had a thorough enough evaluation. More realistically, we define healthy to mean no detectable health problems or symptoms of disease. As we age, we accept minor aches and pains and changes in our habits and still consider ourselves healthy. Stress alters body function but within a limited and normal range. There are good stresses, such as exercise which generally strengthen your body, and bad stresses, such as tension which tend to weaken your body. When you are healthy your body can handle both forms of stress.

Similar to an iceberg, an underlying disease may remain hidden, revealing only a few symptoms that represent the "tip of the disease." For some individuals, health is an illusion because in reality, underlying disease is present but there are no symptoms to indicate its presence. In T.J.'s case, he developed significant coronary artery disease years before his angina and heart attack. His stress test was unable to detect the clogged coronary vessels. This resulted in a false sense of security and health. It is at this stage that routine health maintenance may fail to detect a problem. Fortunately, the danger of permanent harm is generally minimal at this stage.

MODERATE CONCERN In the level of Moderate Concern, illness is usually detectable. However, an individual's symptoms and disease may progress from mild to severe before he or she decides to seek medical care. Each individual has his or her own threshold that must be reached before deciding to seek medical attention. For some, a minor symptom will lead to a call to their doctor, whereas others must be on death's doorstep.

People seek care when their symptoms create enough pain or fear. They usually develop a frame of mind where they believe they should see or speak to a doctor. But for some individuals, health is like a game of craps. They roll the dice against the odds, hoping lady luck will see them through. In T.J.'s case, he entered the level of Moderate Concern, when he developed chest pain while running. He accurately realized that he was out of shape, but inaccurately interpreted his chest pain as indigestion. Silently, T.J.'s coronary arteries had been developing plaque and narrowing over many years. Only when the arteries became critically narrowed and his body was stressed by exercise did he develop his symptoms which were manifest as angina (tightness and pain in the chest while jogging created an increased demand for oxygen to the heart). It is during this stage that most illnesses are still reversible or treatable if a diagnosis, treatment, and preventive health program are instituted.

It is while in the level of Moderate Concern that most people visit their physician. New or worsening symptoms should be taken very seriously and interpreted with a great deal of suspicion. Symptoms are the bodies warning signals that something is wrong. And like the warning light on a dashboard, you can either ignore or deal with symptoms. (Disconnecting the light does not solve the problem.) Your goal in this stage is to receive the care required to circumvent and prevent damage to your body. It may be necessary to be persistent and aggressive regarding your care, especially if your symptoms begin to create a concern that your health may be in danger.

SUBSTANTIAL CONCERN/DANGER In the level of Substantial Concern/ Danger, the person is aware of the pain or the failure of the body to function normally. There is a sense that your health is at risk. This is the stage when the illness can cause irreversible damage to the body. The injury may be minor (a minimal heart attack) or severe (a massive one), but if the disease is treated and detected early enough, a partial or full recovery with a transition back to health may be possible. Exercise 5-2 will help you determine your level of concern about your health and illness.

PREVENTION
The sense of concern is modulated by how much you know about your body. Health awareness can be increased through education, and health maintenance can be improved by practicing prevention.

The key to staying healthy is detecting, treating, and preventing progression of disease before it causes irreversible damage. The later you intervene the greater the risk for permanent damage.

Generally, symptoms are usually minor early in an illness. Unfortunately, the disease may not be detectable with routine preventive examinations and tests. As the disease progresses, the symptoms become more apparent and the doctor's examination and tests usually turn positive. This is why vigilant and repetitive preventive testing is necessary.

It is important not to be lulled into a false sense of security just because a preventive test is interpreted as normal. For example, early in breast cancer, a mammogram may not detect growing cancer cells; the test may be interpreted as normal. If you receive a follow-up mammogram within one year, though, chances are greater that those growing cancer cells will be detected before they metastasize (disseminate into the body, making the cancer more difficult to cure). A simple lumpectomy may cure you. However, if the follow-up mammogram is not performed for two or three years, there is a far greater chance that the cancer will metastasize. Preventive tests and other measures are even more important if you have a suspicious or atypical mammogram or if you have a strong family history of breast cancer. In those situations, the following are strongly advised: early repeat mammograms, routine follow-up exams by your doctor, and monthly self examinations; adherence to a preventive diet; and avoidance of medications that increase your risks for breast cancer. For men, an analogous behavior pattern can apply to prostate cancer. Do your best to practice preventive medicine by eliminating disease when symptoms are minimal—before there is significant bodily damage. The best medicine is prevention.

DO I NEED A DOCTOR?

It is often said that "what you don't know can't hurt you." But in medicine, what you don't know may not only hurt you, it may kill you. Some guidelines to assist you in deciding whether or not you are sick and need to see a doctor are:

1. When you experience a new symptom that is persistent or interfering with your lifestyle, call or see a doctor for an initial checkup.
2. If the symptom persists, get periodic checkups to ensure that a disease is not progressing.

3. If symptoms worsen or if new symptoms develop that you believe may be harmful, call or make an elective appointment.
4. If you feel you are in eminent danger, visit an urgent care center or get emergency care.

Of all the warning signals your body creates:
- Pain and dysfunction are the strongest indicators that you need to take action.
- The more severe the symptoms and the longer they persist, the greater the call to action.

Think of pain and dysfunction as the body's protective security system that monitors changes and is in charge of damage control. Certainly, some individuals can have "silent" heart attacks, while others can experience an excruciatingly painful hangnail. But in general, the severity of the pain is proportional to the potential danger. Severe pain doesn't necessarily mean that you are dying, but it does mean that you need help.

Each person differs in their ability to fight disease. Exercise 5-3 which begins on page 74 will help you determine whether your condition is serious or not. It will also give you an indication of the urgency of your symptoms. Remember you should always immediately call a doctor or go to the emergency room if you experience any of the following*:
- Extreme pain
- Compromise of a necessary bodily function, such as circulation, breathing or mental activity
- Significant trauma
- Ingestion of toxic chemicals

INSIDER'S HINT
If you think you are sick enough to call the doctor and ask for advice, then call.

MAKING DECISIONS
Making good health decisions is not always as easy as it seems. This is illustrated by T.J.'s case. A series of unwise lifestyle choices and

---

*This list is a guideline and does not include all emergencies or symptoms you might have. Each symptom might be important, and if you have any question concerning a symptom, consult your physician.

habits led to an unexpected outcome—heart damage. In retrospect, it is all too easy to see where things went wrong. Although it is difficult to assess symptoms in real time, the key to optimizing your health and getting adequate treatment is recognizing the significance of symptoms before they can cause damage. This can be particularly difficult if the illness accelerates rapidly, as was the case for Jim Henson.

When most living creatures sense danger they instinctively take action to prevent harm to themselves and ensure their survival. Pain, fear, and worry are some of the human "emotional and physical warning signs" that trigger this survival instinct. But, humans can sometimes choose to override and ignore these warning signs.

There is no way in which a lay person can learn enough about medicine so that he or she can always diagnose the cause of their own symptoms. However, there is common sense and experience to guide you. By interpreting your emotional warning signs with balanced reason, you can usually reach the correct decision.

INSIDER'S HINT

It is better to err on the side of caution and see a physician rather than ignore warning signs.

ARE YOU A GAMBLER?

There is always a little bit of Las Vegas involved in the whole process of self assessment. If you have a runny nose and a slight temperature, your bet is that it is a cold. And that is a good bet that you will almost always win. If, however, you bet that your six-week loss of appetite and weight loss is just because you're over stressed at work, then Las Vegas odds are a little different. It is still a good bet that you have a self-limited illness (an illness that will cure itself), but the odds are not quite as good in your favor. If you are losing weight and also have a new lump in your breast, then it would be a bad bet to say that it is just stress.

Discussing your situation with your family and friends may provide you with the needed information to clarify the odds, but this information still will not make your diagnosis a sure thing. Whenever you are deciding whether to seek care, you need to consider if it's worth the gamble.

PRESCRIPTION FOR MAKING GOOD DECISIONS

Knowing when you are sufficiently ill to need a doctor is a matter of good judgment. Although we cannot decide for you when you are sufficiently ill to require a doctor, all variations in your normal health should be regarded with some degree of suspicion. We don't advocate seeing a physician for every little ache or pain, but it is useful to recognize that some molehills can be mountains and some mountains molehills. Remember to ask the questions:

1. Are these symptoms normal or abnormal?
2. How abnormal are these symptoms?
3. How concerned am I about my symptoms?

Then follow these guidelines:

1. Symptoms are the body's warning signals. Pain and dysfunction are the strongest indicators that you need to take action. The more severe the symptoms and the longer they persist the greater the call to action.
2. Your level of concern is your call to action. The greater the concern the greater the call to action.
3. Practice preventive medicine by eliminating disease when symptoms are minimal, before there is any bodily damage.
4. As a general rule, err on the side of caution. If you think you are sick enough to call the doctor and ask for advice, call.

Exercise 5-4 is a summary exercise that will help you to determine whether you need to call a doctor.

EXERCISE 5-1

What Is Your Normal Health Status?

This exercise will help you to establish your normal state of being. Keep this exercise with your personal medical records, so that you can refer back to it when you think your normal state has changed. Also consider updating this exercise each year to record natural changes in your normal state.

ENERGY/ACTIVITY LEVEL

What is your level of energy?

0	1	2	3	4	5	6	7	8	9	10
none		poor		fair			good		excellent	

How often do you exercise per week? _____

What type(s) of exercise do you participate in? _____

_____

_____

Do you experience more energy in the morning, afternoon, or evening?

_____

STRESS LEVEL

How would you rate the current level of stress in your life?

0	1	2	3	4	5	6	7	8	9	10
no stress		mild		moderate		high			intense	

WORK

How many hours do you work in a normal day? _____

SLEEP ACTIVITY

How many hours do you typically sleep per day? _____

How would you describe the quality of your sleep?

terrible   poor   fair   good

ALCOHOL & CIGARETTE USAGE

How many alcoholic drinks do you consume per day _____

or per week _____

How many cigarettes do you smoke per day_____

EXERCISE 5-1

What Is Your Normal Health Status? *(cont.)*

BASIC METABOLISM
For each category write down your normal state.

Morning (basal) temperature:_____

Resting pulse: _____

Blood pressure: _____

SENSES
For each category circle that which currently applies to you.

Vision:

| clear | clear with prescribed correction | mildly impaired | severely impaired |

Hearing:

| good | trouble with quiet sounds | mildly impaired | severely impaired |

URINATION HABITS
For each category circle that which currently applies to you.

Color: pale yellow   dark yellow   cloudy

Frequency: every hour   1–3 hours   3–6 hours

At night: none   1–2   3–4   over 4 times

BOWEL MOVEMENTS
For each category circle that which currently applies to you.

Number per day: 0–1   2–3   4–5   over 5

Color: brown   black   yellow

Character: hard   firm   loose   watery

ADDITIONAL COMMENTS

_____

_____

_____

EXERCISE 5-2

What is Your Level of Concern?

For each level, answer the questions with a "Yes" or "No." Your level of concern will change over time, so complete this exercise periodically.

MINIMAL OR NO CONCERN

_____ Do you generally feel healthy?

_____ Are you without any visible signs or symptoms of illness?

_____ Are you experiencing minor aches, pains, or bodily changes within your normal state?

_____ Are you satisfied with your current health status?

_____ **Number of "Yes" answers**

MODERATE CONCERN

_____ Do you feel that your health is moderately impaired?

_____ Do you notice any visible signs or symptoms of illness?

_____ Are your bodily functions outside of your normal healthy state?

_____ Are you worried about your current health status?

_____ **Number of "Yes" answers**

SUBSTANTIAL CONCERN/DANGER

_____ Do you feel that your health is severely impaired?

_____ Have others noticed and commented on visible signs or symptoms of illness?

_____ Is your body functioning abnormally, and is this impacting your ability to perform daily routines?

_____ Do you sense a "real" danger about your health status?

_____ **Number of "Yes" answers**

SCORING

Total your number of "Yes" answers for each level of concern. Rate yourself according to the following scale:

1 "Yes" answer in a level: your health status does not reflect this level of concern.

2 "Yes" answers in a level: your health status moderately reflects this level of concern.

3-4 "Yes" answers in a level: your health status strongly reflects this level of concern. If you have 3 or 4 "Yes" answers in either the Moderate Concern level or Substantial Concern/Danger level, you should contact your physician to schedule an appointment and discuss your concerns.

Your Current Level of Pain and Dysfunction

This exercise will help you to decide if you need to see a doctor. The following rating scales and questions will help you to understand and assess your current symptoms. Symptoms are the body's warning signals. Pain and dysfunction (the change in how the body works) are the strongest indicators that you need to take action. The more severe the symptoms and the longer they persist, the greater the need for you to take action.

LEVEL OF PAIN

Where on your body is the pain located? Using the diagram at right, indicate with an X where you are feeling pain.

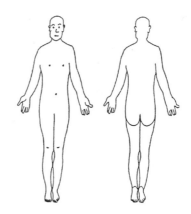

What is your current level of pain?

0	1	2	3	4	5	6	7	8	9	10
no pain		mild		moderate		severe		intense		excruciating

How long have you experienced this pain?_____

Has your pain felt better than your current level?   Y   N

What is your best level? _____

When did you last feel this good?_____

EXERCISE 5-3

Your Current Level of Pain and Dysfunction *(cont.)*

Has your pain felt worse than your current level?   Y   N

What is your worst level? _____

When did you last feel this bad? _____

What level of pain could you live with on a daily basis? _____

LEVEL OF DYSFUNCTION

What part of your body is dysfunctional? _____

Using the diagram at right, indicate with an X where you are dysfunctional.

What is your current level
of dysfunction?

0	1	2	3	4	5	6	7	8	9	10
no dysfunction		mild	moderate		severe		very severe			life-altering

How long have you experienced this dysfunction? _____

Has your dysfunction felt better than your current level? Y   N

What is your best level of dysfunction? _____

When did you last feel this good? _____

Has your dysfunction felt worse than your current level? Y   N

What is your worst level of dysfunction? _____

When did you last feel this bad? _____

What level of dysfunction could you live with on a daily basis? ____

EXERCISE 5-4

Do You Really Need a Doctor?

Your level of concern over any pain and dysfunction is your call to action. The greater the concern, the greater the call to action.

What is your current level of pain?

0	1	2	3	4	5	6	7	8	9	10
no pain		mild		moderate		severe		intense		excruciating

What is your current level of dysfunction?

0	1	2	3	4	5	6	7	8	9	10
no dysfunction		mild		moderate		severe		very severe		life-altering

What is your current overall level of concern?

0	1	2	3	4	5	6	7	8	9	10
none			minimal			moderate			substantial	

You can practice preventive medicine by eliminating disease when symptoms are minimal, that is, before there is any bodily damage.

Are you suffering from bodily damage?   Y   N

If yes, what is your damage? _____

If no, what are your reasons to believe you have no damage? _____

_____

As a general rule, it is usually better to err on the side of caution. If you think you are sick enough to call the doctor and ask for advice, then call!

Do you think you are sick enough to call a doctor?   Y   N

Take this exercise with you to the doctor to help explain your symptoms.

_____

_____

_____

_____

_____

_____

Chapter 6

Finding the Right Kind of Doctor for Your Illness

For a month or so John had been experiencing a decreased appetite, stomach pains, and a full feeling while he ate. Even his coworkers had noticed his pale appearance and weight loss. Despite moving to Seattle from college five years earlier, John still did not have a doctor. He had been healthy and never really needed one—until now.

John knew his problem wasn't an emergency, so he asked acquaintances for advice. His roommate only knew a psychiatrist, and his boss could only suggest her gynecologist. They weren't likely to help, so John opened the Yellow Pages, closed his eyes, and pointed a finger.

Soon he was in Dr. Oldguys' waiting room, sitting next to two octogenarians reading *Modern Maturity*. It finally dawned on him, maybe he should have looked up the word geriatrician before making his appointment. But he had already taken a day off from work, rearranged his week's schedule, and driven 45 minutes to get there. By the time it was his turn to see the doctor, John realized that he could have done a better job finding the right doctor. Perhaps the visit wouldn't be a total loss, though, if he could at least get a referral to someone who could help him with his problem.

CONCERNED ABOUT FINDING THE RIGHT DOCTOR?

You've determined that you need to see a doctor. The next step is to find the right doctor. With diligence and patience the chances are good that you will find a doctor who can meet your medical and personality needs. This chapter will help you assess which type of doctor is correct for you, and advise you on how and where to find that doctor.

TYPES OF PHYSICIANS

PRIMARY CARE PHYSICIANS

These doctors provide for your basic health care needs, and are most likely the first to address any problems you might have. These doctors provide most of the basic medical services including preventive care and initial diagnosis and treatment of common illnesses. A primary care doctor treats common ailments and coordinates complex care.

The most common types of traditional Western Medicine primary care physicians are:

FAMILY/GENERAL PRACTITIONERS treat both adults and children for a wide range of medical, surgical, and obstetric/gynecologic conditions. These physicians may have either an M.D. or D.O. degree.

PEDIATRICIANS treat children under age 18.

INTERNISTS treat adults for a wide range of medical conditions.

OBSTETRICIAN-GYNECOLOGISTS provide primary care to female adult patients, and in special cases, may treat illnesses other than women's health problems.

SPECIALISTS

Specialists have additional training in specific areas of medical practice. They have extensive knowledge and experience regarding specific diseases and their treatments. A specialist is someone who you may visit for a brief interval for a procedure or second opinion or for a long period of time for a chronic problem that requires specialist expertise. There are four subgroups of specialists.

INTERNAL MEDICINE SPECIALISTS are trained in general internal medicine followed by additional training in a particular sub-specialty area. For example, cardiology (heart disease), gastroenterology (digestive organs), and pulmonary specialists (lungs).

MEDICINE SPECIALISTS have trained for one year in general medicine and then spent two to four years in residency training specializing in specific disciplines such as neurology (nervous system), psychiatry (emotions), or dermatology (skin).

DIAGNOSTICIANS have trained for one year in general medicine and then spent two to four years in residency training specializing in specific diagnostic disciplines such as radiology (x-ray doctors) or pathology (laboratory medicine doctors).

SURGEONS spend three to five years in residency training learning medicine and surgery.

Appendix 1 provides more information on the various specialties. This list will help you sort through the Greek and Latin names that are used in the medical profession to define different specialties.

WHO SHOULD YOU SEE? THE GENERALIST OR SPECIALIST OR BOTH?

Medical technology and knowledge have expanded at a terrific rate. As a result you may require more than one doctor. A family/general practitioner should be competently able to handle an extremely wide range of common problems, but complex problems or intricate procedures are best dealt with by specialists.

If you know or suspect your diagnosis, it may be appropriate for you to go directly to a specialist. If you choose to see a specialist first, you will need to decide which type to see. If it is obvious that your symptoms involve one main area, such as lungs or intestines, then you use Appendix 1 to find the right specialist.

Some specialists do not see patients who are self referred (patient calls the doctor directly) or who do not have a primary care physician. This is done to avoid visits from people who may not be appropriate for that specialist's particular specialty. Also, many specialists do not wish to become a patient's general medical doctor by default if other medical problems develop. Given the inherent narrow focus of specialists, most do not feel comfortable performing functions normally done by primary care physicians. As a result, a specialist may require that you be evaluated initially by a generalist. Or, she may want to ensure that you have a primary care physician who can treat problems that might arise outside of the specialist's area of expertise.

COORDINATING YOUR CARE

It's best to have a generalist—a family physician or internal medicine physician—who can coordinate your care in order to avoid duplicate treatments and/or medications that interfere or interact adversely with each other. Seeing only specialists for specific problems may fragment your care. If you see one doctor for your arthritis, one for your heart, one for your toe nail infection, one for your allergies, and one for your ulcer, you may get lost in the maze. Your specialists may not be aware that you are being treated by others.

If you do not have a generalist "coordinator," then you will have to assume the responsibility of coordinating your own care. However, this can prove risky to your health, as illustrated by the story of Don Peters.

Don injured his lower leg. A week later he developed a blood clot that broke off and traveled to his lung. He responded well to treatment, but needed to be on a blood thinner for the next six months. Two months after the accident, while working in his yard, he injured his back. He decided to see an orthopedist, a specialist in back pain, for this problem rather than his internist. Only a brief history and physical were performed. Don was diagnosed with back strain and prescribed an anti-inflammatory medicine. Three weeks later, Don showed up in the ER after several days of black stools and abdominal pain. He had developed a bleeding ulcer because of taking an anti-inflammatory while on a blood thinner.

Two major mistakes occurred here. Don didn't tell his orthopedist he was on a blood thinner, and the orthopedist didn't ask! It is OK to see more than one physician, especially if you have a set of complicated problems. However, it is important that someone oversees your care. Making sure that the right hand acts in concert with the left is essential for not only getting the best treatment but also avoiding injury because of conflicting treatments.

Think of your health care as a giant construction project. The general contractor has overall control of the building but delegates specific projects to experts. Wiring goes to the electricians, pipes to the plumbers, and duct work to sheet metal workers. If you go to a series of specialists, we recommend that you have a generalist who coordinates your care and ensures that all the pieces fit correctly.

ANCILLARY PROVIDERS

Nurse midwives, nurse practitioners, occupational therapists, physical therapists, physician assistants, psychologists, social workers, and others function as part of the traditional health care team. Psychologists have always worked independently, but the others have usually worked under the guidance of a physician. Over the past several years patients have had more direct access to many of these providers than they have had in the past. In Appendix 1 you will find more detailed definitions of these different types of providers.

ALTERNATIVE MEDICINE PROVIDERS

Alternative to what? Traditionally health care has been provided by medical doctors (M.D.) and osteopathic doctors (D.O.). Over the years, though, people with other training have also sought to provide primary and specialty care to patients. Acupuncturists, chiropractors, herbalists, homeopaths, massage therapists, and naturopaths, to name a few, are usually considered alternative medical providers. (On page 315 you will find a list of these alternative care specialties.)

Should you use an alternative medical provider? This is a personal decision. Many people turn to alternative medicine when they have not improved with traditional care. Others seek alternative therapy first because of a bad experience with traditional medicine or a general distrust of the medical establishment. Some patients choose alternative medicine because it is less invasive and in some cases less expensive. There is no right answer as to what you should do; the answer depends upon your preferences and philosophies. (This is further discussed in Chapter 12.)

All too often, "traditional" Western medicine has considered alternative medicine as less scientific and not effective. But many novel and currently accepted treatments in traditional medicine once fell within the domain of alternative medicine. Acupuncture, massage therapy, and high-dose vitamin supplementation are but a few of the alternative therapies that, once ridiculed, now are gaining acceptance from traditional medical establishment. In fact, the government has recently begun to increase the funds appropriated for alternative medicine research.

For many people, alternative medicine embodies aspects of care not emphasized by traditional western methods. First, there is the perception that alternative medicine is natural and safer than western medicine which is considered synthetic and potentially more dangerous. Second, there is the sense that patients control their care and medical destiny to a greater degree in alternative medicine. In part, this feeling may be derived from the belief that the patient is more involved in alternative medicine. Finally, alternative medicine seems to direct more of its focus on improving everyday living by applying wellness techniques that reduce stress (meditation) and improve the body's energy (yoga and aromatic therapy).

If you see an alternative provider, you should be aware of some pitfalls.

- There are alternative practitioners who lack the necessary skills and training to diagnosis serious illnesses. A delay in diagnosis may result in severe complications.
- Most alternative treatments have not been scientifically tested with the same scrutiny as traditional medicine. Using an unproven remedy may increase your risk of disease progression. Also, there is a difference between feeling better for the short term and being effectively treated or cured in the long term.
- Some alternative providers are "unregulated," and there may be no independent method to establish competence and effectiveness.
- Vitamins, alternative medicines, and herbs can have serious side effects.

If you choose an alternative provider, we believe that a combination of traditional and alternative medicine probably provides the best system of checks and balances. Additionally, you should regularly assess your response to treatment. If you do this, you will be less likely to waste precious time and money on traditional or alternative therapies that do not work. Positive results are the best measure of success.

If you feel consistently better with treatment over a prolonged period of time and the treatment is not harmful, then you are probably getting value. If not, going back week after week for ineffective treatments does not make sense. This is true whether you are seeing an alternative or traditional provider. Despite the best of intentions, a bad result is still a bad result.

INSIDER'S HINT

If you choose an alternative provider, we believe that a combination of traditional and alternative medicine probably provides the best system of checks and balances.

OTHER SOURCES OF CARE

There are two other commonly used sources of care, which have advantages and disadvantages.

EMERGENCY ROOMS (ERS) *Advantages:* Trained personnel 24 hours a day, 7 days a week; no appointment is needed; equipped to handle serious life-threatening problems immediately.

Disadvantages: Expensive; may need to wait a long time before being seen; there is no consistent follow-up care.

URGENT CARE CENTERS (DOC-IN-THE-BOX) *Advantages:* Extended hours, usually 7 A.M. to 10 P.M.; no appointment is needed; usually have a lab and x-ray facility on site for quick test results; trained to handle problems that are not serious enough to warrant a trip to the ER but which can't wait for a routine office visit; less expensive than an ER; may offer routine follow-up care and may provide primary care services.

Disadvantages: Less likely to offer as complete a range of services as a primary care doctor; often you will not be able to see the same doctor in follow-up; do not provide 24 hour coverage nor do they admit patients to the hospital, so another doctor would need to take over your care.

WHAT ARE YOUR DOCTOR'S QUALIFICATIONS?

Did your brain surgeon graduate from a non-accredited foreign medical school, then do his residency through a mail order correspondence course offered on the back of a matchbook cover? Most likely not. But it would be nice to know something about the qualifications required of your doctor to whom you will entrust your health.

Typical physician training includes:
- 4 years of college
- 4 years of medical school
- 1 year of hospital apprenticeship-like training, called an internship. Interns are M.D.s but they cannot practice on their own. After this internship and after passing the National Boards, a doctor qualifies as a general practitioner and can get a license to practice medicine.
- 2 to 5 years of additional hospital-based training known as residency. Residents are supervised by other more senior residents and by attending doctors. Attending Physicians are practicing doctors who choose to teach at universities or teaching hospitals. By the final or senior year of residency, a doctor is functioning almost independently. The overseeing

and most senior resident is called the chief resident. Upon completing residency, and passing a specialty board exam, the doctor is considered a fully functioning Diplomat of that specialty (for example, Family Practice, Pediatrician, Neurologist, Dermatologist, General Surgeon, General Internist).

• Several additional years in a fellowship or subspecialty training. The fellow studies a specific organ system or disease in ever greater detail than the resident (for example, heart—cardiologist, stomach and intestines—gastroenterologist, and joints and immune system—rheumatologist). General surgeons are capable of doing many abdominal, chest, and extremity surgeries, but a subspecialist surgeon (for example, a vascular or cardio-thoracic surgeon) will seek additional training beyond general surgery to concentrate on specific types of surgery. At the end of subspecialty another exam is often required to become a Diplomat of the subspecialty.

BOARDS, LICENSES, AND CREDENTIALS

In order to be licensed to practice medicine, a doctor must pass the national boards, a two-part examination with part one taken in medical school and part two after internship, or the FLEX examination, specifically given to foreign medical school graduates. Some states also require that state boards be passed.

After internship training is completed, in order to practice medicine in your state the doctor must obtain a medical license from the state. No real competence is required to obtain a license. The state license must be renewed yearly and is a requirement for malpractice insurance. Most states require a doctor to complete a specified amount of continuing medical education (CME) in order to be relicensed.

After internship, most physicians complete a residency, such as pediatrics, internal medicine, family practice, general surgery, and many physicians complete advanced training in subspecialty areas called fellowships. After completing these programs, doctors can take board certification examinations. Physicians who pass these tests are allowed to advertise that they are "board certified" in a given discipline, which indicates an accepted level of competence in their field.

The most direct way to determine your doctor's credentials is to ask him about his training and CME. Other options would be to look on his walls for diplomas and certificates, or ask to see a copy of his curriculum vitae (cv).

DOES IT MATTER WHERE YOUR DOCTOR TRAINED?

Many factors determine where a person attends medical school. Excellent practicing physicians may come out of both Harvard and a small lesser known state medical school. Perhaps a better indicator of skill is where the physician did his internship, residency, or fellowship. Then again, maybe not. A doctor who did his residency at a smaller and lesser known hospital could be just as good as someone who trained at Johns Hopkins. Once you have established your doctor's basic competence, your personal preference usually is more of an overriding factor than which medical school or residency program your doctor attended.

WHAT IS THE DOCTOR'S STANDING IN THE COMMUNITY?

This may be difficult but not impossible to ascertain. Licenses and recertification reveal a basic level of competence. In smaller communities, reputations can be made or broken in relatively short times. Speak to friends, relatives, neighbors, or other patients and see what you can find out. There is a simple principle in customer service: If good service is provided, other people may be aware of it. If terrible service is given, everyone hears about it. If you hear many negative reports about your prospective doctor, beware. State and medical societies, the state licensing bureau, and the Better Business Bureau can inform you about a health care giver's standing in the community.

WHAT FACTORS ARE IMPORTANT TO YOU IN FINDING A DOCTOR?

Before you begin your search, it is important for you to think about what factors will influence your selection. For instance, your friend needs a gynecologist. She asks you for advice. You give her the name of your ob/gyn, Jack Doe. You like him and find him to be quite good. Your friend thanks you politely, but doesn't take his telephone number. You are puzzled. Why didn't she want to see your ob/gyn? Possibly she wants a female doctor, or one that is closer to her work or home. Different people have different needs. Exercise 6-1 will help you to determine which factors are important, and ultimately help you select the right doctor .

SOURCES OF INFORMATION TO HELP YOU FIND A DOCTOR

If you do not have a primary care physician to evaluate you or to help you find a specialist, you will need to consider the following available sources of information about the doctors in your community.

DOCTORS YOU'VE SEEN IN THE PAST. Does that doctor deal with the kinds of symptoms you are having?

GROUP PRACTICES. Several physicians work together in a single or group of offices. If you know a good doctor is in a group but not taking new patients, consider going to one of the partners. Doctors prefer working with other doctors who share a similar level of competence.

FAMILY AND FRIENDS. They are in tune to your needs and personality. You should be critical of the information provided. Do you respect their opinions and behaviors in general? If yes, listening makes sense.

SUPPORT GROUPS THAT SPECIALIZE IN YOUR ILLNESS. Many disease-specific support groups hold meetings regularly at local hospitals, community centers, churches, etc. Members of these groups usually spend a lot of time in finding the physicians that can most satisfy their needs. Ask about the group's experiences and who they would recommend.

NON-PROFIT ORGANIZATIONS AND FOUNDATIONS. These organizations include the American Diabetes Association, The American Cancer Society, the Arthritis Foundation, etc.

THE LOCAL HOSPITAL. The medical staff office will give you a list of physicians on staff and their areas of expertise, along with office telephone numbers.

THE HOSPITAL STAFF. Nurses are usually in a good position to see who delivers the best care in the hospital. It is then reasonable to extrapolate this to outside of the hospital. Try a friendly conversation in the cafeteria or at the nursing station.

ER INSTRUCTION. When seen and discharged from the ER, you may be given the name of an outpatient doctor for follow-up.

STATE AND COUNTY MEDICAL SOCIETIES. These organizations, composed of physicians in each county and the state, offer educational programs, perform lobbying functions, act as official "police officers" of the profession, and serve as ombudsmen in handling patients' complaints.

These medical societies frequently have referral lists. Though they cannot specifically endorse any particular doctor, they can tell you who is available in your area. County and State societies are most easily found by looking in the *Yellow Pages* under "Physicians & Surgeons-Referral & Information."

THE TELEPHONE BOOK. A phone book search will let you know who practices in your town or community but little more than this unless the doctor has a larger advertisement.

1-800-FIND-A-DOC. Some cities and towns now have telephone services to assist you in gathering this information. They can be found in the *Yellow Pages* under "Physicians & Surgeons- Referral & Information." These services may be independently run enterprises in which physicians pay a small fee to be in the services' database or they can be run by local hospitals or state medical associations. These services are usually designed to drum up business, not to help you make critical decisions about your best source for care.

THE INTERNET. The Internet may be an excellent source to find a physician, especially if you have a rare illness or if your illness has baffled local experts. Communicating with others in the chat rooms may direct you to other individuals dealing with similar problems. You may find home pages on particular diseases by support groups, treatment organizations, or other patients. It also helps to check the Internet for the experts who are writing medical journal articles about your condition. Consider calling, emailing, or writing that expert doctor and asking if he or she can recommend anyone to you who practices in your area. See if any of the doctors writing articles are from your area. Remember, information on the Internet is not censored and must be reviewed with a "large grain of salt." Chapter 4 discusses the Internet and how to use it.

FINDING A DOCTOR IN ANOTHER CITY

You can call your hometown doctor just as if you were home. Your doctor may be able to call a prescription in to a nearby pharmacy (except for narcotics). Be prepared to have the number of the local pharmacy available when you call. Your doctor may request that you come in for a follow-up visit as soon as you get home. If he cannot diagnose you over the phone, or if the problem sounds serious, he may ask that you be evaluated further by a local physician. First, ask your doctor for his advice on whom to see. He may be able to recommend someone.

When you call for the appointment, use your hometown doctor's name and explain the circumstances of your situation. Other options are to get help from the friend, client, or business associate that you are visiting; ask the hotel concierge; or use one of the other options discussed in the preceding section. If you are overseas, there are a number of organizations that provide worldwide medical assistance. Their services vary from being able to make appointments for you to helping you find emergency medical care. These organizations charge fees that vary according to the services they provide. Some of these organizations are listed here:

- U.S. State Department Citizen's Emergency Care—
  (202) 647-5225
- International Association for Medical Assistance to
  Travelers—(716) 754-4883
- International SOS—(215) 244-1500 or (800) 523-8930
- AirAmbulance Network—(305) 447-0458 or
  (800) 327-1966
- Hoteldocs—(800) HOTELDR

CALLING MEDICAL MECCA

We all want the best medical care. At times we may believe that the best care can only be administered by an "expert," someone at a secondary downtown referral hospital or a tertiary university hospital—so-called medical meccas.

The easiest and recommended way to be seen by an expert physician practicing at one of these facilities is to ask your treating physician for a referral, preferably to someone he knows that has a reputation for being the "best." If this is not possible, alternative sources for learning about experts include; friends, magazine articles, the Internet, and the library. Medical librarians are an exceptionally good resource for helping you facilitate your search for an expert.

Sometimes, smaller meccas may not provide you with the answers or treatment you desire, especially if you have an extremely rare disease. If that is the case, then you may need to travel to one of the national or even international meccas such as The Mayo Clinic.

LAST-MINUTE QUESTIONS TO CONSIDER

It is difficult and frustrating knowing whether the doctor you have chosen is good or even treating your condition in the best possible way. For instance, a doctor who can do excellent surgery of the lower back (lumbar spine) may not be as good at operating on the upper spine (cervical spine). There are several questions that may help you in knowing what you are getting. Ask your doctor:

1. How many of these procedures have you done this year? In your career? How many patients with this condition have you treated this year? In your career?

2. What center in the city, state, or in the country treats the most patients with my condition? On average, how many patients with my condition do they see each year? (You may wish to call that institution and get a second opinion.)

3. Who would you go to if you had the same condition? (Ask if she would set up a second opinion appointment with that individual.)

ARE YOU FREE TO CHOOSE?

You can see any health care professional you want as long as he or she is willing to see you, but health care professionals are under no obligation to provide you with an appointment.

Your insurance company will most likely have a say in who you can see. The first part of the process of finding a doctor is to check with your subscriber information and find out if you have a restricted list of physicians from which to choose. Please refer to Chapter 14, regarding insurance and physician choice issues.

EXERCISE 6-1

Selecting a Doctor

This exercise lists some of the generally asked questions about doctors. You have the right to this information so that you can make an informed choice in physicians. There are several ways in which you can obtain this information: 1) Ask your doctor directly, 2) Ask your doctor's staff, 3) Review the diplomas in your doctor's office, 4) Conduct a literature or name search on the Internet, or 5) Contact your state medical society (look in the *Yellow Pages* under "Physicians & Surgeons-Referral & Information" for the societies' telephone numbers).

GENERAL CHARACTERISTICS

1. Name of physician: _____

2. Sex of physician: male_____   female_____

3. Age of physician: _____

PROFESSIONAL QUALIFICATIONS

1. Where did the doctor go to medical school? _____

2. Is the doctor licensed to practice?:   Y   N

3. Is the doctor board certified?:   Y   N

4. Did the doctor do specialized training?:   Y   N

In what?: _____

5. Is the doctor fellowship certified?:   Y   N

In what?: _____

6. Has the doctor taught at a university?:   Y   N

Where?:_____

7. Has the doctor done any medical research
or published any papers?:   Y   N

In what?: _____

(Note: You can go to the library and review their publications if you are curious.)

Selecting a Doctor *(cont.)*

8. Has the doctor ever been disciplined
by a medical society?:   Y   N

a. If so, for what?: _____

b. For how long?:_____

9. Has the doctor ever been sued for malpractice?:   Y   N

a. If so, for what?: _____

b. What happened?: _____
(Note: In this era, most physicians have been sued. And if they
haven't, they will be sued. This is no longer as significant a question
as it was 15 years ago. But you still owe it to yourself to find out what
happened and why.)

10. Has the doctor ever had his license suspended?:   Y   N

Why?_____

11. Has the doctor ever had hospital privileges
suspended or revoked?:   ˊ   Y   N

a. Why? _____

b. For how long?:_____

12. Has the doctor ever been convicted of a felony?: Y   N

a. For what?_____

LOCATION AND CONVENIENCE

1. Is the doctor's office close to work or home?:   Y   N

2. Is the doctor's office close to the hospital?:   Y   N

3. What are the office hours? _____

4. Is the doctor on call?:   Y   N

5. How does the doctor handle emergency situations?_____

_____

_____

Chapter 7

Getting Organized for Your Appointment

Five years ago, Sam was diagnosed as having ulcerative colitis. For the first three years, his disease was under excellent control. A job promotion brought him to a new city, though, and he began experiencing a recurrence of his ulcerative colitis symptoms (possibly provoked by the stress of moving and a new job). Sam had not visited a doctor in the new town, but he had been given the name of a good gastrointestinal (GI) specialist by his hometown doctor.

Sam made an appointment but forgot to write down directions to the doctor's office. As a result, he arrived late to the appointment. However, the office personnel were understanding and reshuffled the schedule to accommodate him. As Sam checked in for his appointment, the receptionist asked if he had remembered to get a referral note and collect his old medical records from his former primary care doctor. Sam had forgotten. Without those details, the GI specialist could only make an educated guess as to what combination of medications would work best for Sam.

To make matters worse, when the bill arrived four weeks later for the visit, Sam was surprised to learn that because he had failed to get a referral, he was responsible for all of the charges—not his insurance company. After many letters and phone calls, Sam did receive partial reimbursement. And over the course of the next few months, through trial and error, he found a primary care physician he liked. Still, he could not help but think, "There must be a better, less stressful way to make an appointment with a doctor."

There is!

INSIDER'S HINT
....
The keys to obtaining optimal health care are preparation, organization, and prioritization.

WHAT KIND OF AN APPOINTMENT SHOULD YOU MAKE?

Before you make an appointment you need to know what kind of appointment to make.

FIRST VISIT. A first visit with a generalist/primary care provider for basic health care is typically an overview of the patient's health and an introduction of the patient and physician to each other. The first visit with a specialist generally focuses on a relatively narrow range of problems and complaints. The scope of a first visit can vary greatly from simply getting acquainted to a comprehensive evaluation. First visits usually will last 30 to 60 minutes. During this visit, the doctor obtains a complete medical history and performs a physical exam. Diagnostic laboratory and x-ray testing may also be ordered at the visit's completion.

FOLLOW-UP VISIT. The two main reasons for follow-up visits are: 1) ongoing routine health maintenance, including minor ailments, and 2) continued assessment and treatment for complex illnesses. During follow-up visits, test results and treatment plans are discussed. Additional testing may be ordered. A follow-up visit can also be used to present new problems that may have occurred since the last visit. Follow-up visits are usually shorter than first visits and range from 5 to 30 minutes.

REFERRAL VISIT. This visit occurs when a physician requests that a patient see another health care provider. Most commonly, a generalist will refer the patient to a specialist either to render an opinion or to assume control of a particular aspect of his or her care.

ARRANGING YOUR APPOINTMENT

Whether you are revisiting your life long family doctor or seeing someone for the first time, you should be prepared and organized before you pick-up the telephone and dial. It is easy to become flustered and forgetful when not prepared.

INSIDER'S HINT

Organization reduces anxiety.

Once you are on the telephone, remember to address these key points.

This may be obvious, but SCHEDULE AN APPOINTMENT YOU CAN KEEP. If you miss the appointment or cancel less than 24 hours prior to the appointment, some physicians may charge a fee which may be as much as the complete cost of the visit. Mark the appointment immediately into your calendar. This way you won't forget it or have to call the doctor's office to reconfirm the time or date.

AVOID ASKING FOR THE FIRST AND LAST APPOINTMENTS OF THE DAY. These times are in greatest demand given the busy work and school schedules of many people.

ASK FOR DIRECTIONS TO THE OFFICE AND PARKING INSTRUCTIONS IF NECESSARY.

ASK FOR PRE-APPOINTMENT INSTRUCTIONS. You may not be able to eat or drink before your appointment because your doctor may perform lab work which requires you to fast. This may even include a glass of water or a vitamin pill.

ASK IF YOU WILL NEED ASSISTANCE IN GETTING HOME. You could be given a sedative during an outpatient procedure or eyedrops to dilate your eyes during an exam. Also, you might have some minor surgery or procedure done to a part of your body that limits its normal use. If any of these circumstances apply or you are given anything that impairs your ability to drive, then you need to arrange for someone to drive you home from your visit. Exercise 7-1 is a checklist of items you will need for making an appointment.

It doesn't hurt to call and reconfirm your appointment, though the physician's office will probably call you—especially if you are scheduled for a new patient visit, which typically lasts an hour. They will want to make sure that an hour of the doctor's time will not go wasted, particularly if there is a long wait for first patient visits. Also this gives them the opportunity to remind you of special instructions or give advice on how to prepare for your appointment. It is less likely that you will be called for a follow-up visit but certainly not unheard of. If you have the slightest concern about not being able to keep the date or time of your appointment give the doctor's office a call, as far in advance as possible.

ARE GET-ACQUAINTED VISITS AVAILABLE?

A get-acquainted visit can help you to reaffirm your decision to see one physician over another. However, these types of visits are not always available. Different policies exist in different doctor's practices and in different geographic areas. Specialties that deal in plastic surgery and infertility problems usually do offer these types of visits. However, a general practitioner is less likely to have the time for a get-acquainted visit. Additionally, you will have to pay for a get-acquainted visit out of your own pocket. If a physician does not offer a get-acquainted visit, do not necessarily hold that against her. She may be just the right doctor for you.

ARRANGING A REFERRAL VISIT

If you are trying to schedule an appointment with a new doctor, then you will need to have the name and phone number of the referring doctor, as well as the reason for the referral. You may need your primary care physician to send a referral letter. You also might want to request a copy of the referral from your primary care physician to bring with you to your appointment. This could help you to avoid bureaucratic problems. Additionally, it is usually wise to maintain copies of referral letters in your own personal medical records.

It is also advisable to inform your insurance carrier or managed care program about the need for a referral. If prior authorization for the referral is required, calling may save you money and hassles. If you do need authorization and you don't call, then you will most likely end up paying for the appointment out of your own pocket—a costly mistake.

INSIDER'S HINT

When in doubt, call your insurance company for prior authorization. It could save you money.

For some specialists, waiting times for appointments may be weeks to months. If no appointment is available in the near future, and your situation is urgent but not an emergency, then you may need to call your primary care physician to intervene on your behalf. She might be able to get you an appointment either before or after regular office hours or even during the specialist's lunch hour. If your situation is not urgent, then ask to be put on a cancellation list. Appointment slots may become available during the week as other patients cancel. If this is the case, just remember that you might have to see the specialist at a time that is not convenient for you.

WHEN IS IT APPROPRIATE TO CANCEL AN APPOINTMENT?

Observe how you feel between the time you make the appointment and the time you actually go to the doctor. If you feel worse, you might need to call and move the appointment up if possible. However, if you feel better, then consider whether you are really all better or just improved. Keeping a medical log (diary) may give you a more concrete idea as to whether you are getting better or worse. (Exercise 9-2 on page 129 gives you information on how to maintain a medical log of your office visits and telephone calls.) Call your doctor right away if you want to cancel an appointment. But make sure it's for the right reason; you truly do not need medical attention. Convincing yourself that you are at 100 percent, when in truth you are not, may cause harm and delay important medical treatment.

Scheduling Your Appointment

Before scheduling your appointment, the following items are useful:
- pencil/pen
- calendar
- paper
- list of questions

The following is information that you will usually provide to the receptionist. Write it down here, so that you will have it available when you schedule your appointment.

Name of your primary care doctor:_____

Name and phone number of your insurance company: _____

Your plan number: _____

Your group insurance number if applicable: _____

Your individual subscriber number: _____

Disabilities or special needs, such as an interpreter or the need to bring

a surrogate decision maker:_____

_____

List any additional questions you need to ask the receptionist:

1._____

2._____

3._____

4._____

Remember to get the following information from the receptionist: directions and special instructions to prepare for the appointment (such as no foods or fluids before the appointment).

_____

_____

_____

_____

_____

_____

Chapter 8

Preparing Your Medical History

It just wasn't Sam's day. If you recall, in the last chapter we met Sam when he was having a bad day—he had ulcerative colitis. Not only had Sam been late to his doctor's appointment and forgotten to bring some important information, but he also failed to bring a list of medications he was currently taking—and had taken in the past—for the colitis.

Unfortunately, this lack of preparation somewhat compromised Sam's evaluation. The appointment took longer than normal and Sam needed to return in three weeks for another one, this time with his medical documents. The GI specialist provided Sam with a prescription but the doctor wasn't as confident in his medical treatment plan as he would have been if he had had Sam's records.

This chapter focuses on preparing the information you will need to get the most out of a doctor's appointment.

WHAT INFORMATION SHOULD YOU BRING WITH YOU?

A patient's relationship with a doctor is similar to that of a computer and its user. You must first provide your doctor with accurate information so that he can make a correct diagnosis and devise an effective treatment plan. And just like a computer, if you provide the doctor with useless or limited information, you won't get a full answer.

INSIDER'S HINT
Accurate information leads to a correct diagnosis which leads to effective treatment.

WRITE DOWN YOUR CHIEF COMPLAINTS, SYMPTOMS, AND SIGNS. *Chief complaints,* as you can guess, are just that—your main ailments or concerns. These are what have prompted you to see your doctor in the first place. You might be surprised how many people never get around to talking to their doctor about their chief complaint during a visit. That's why it's important to clarify in your mind your most pressing concerns.

In the medical world, the chief complaint is a product of symptoms and signs. *Symptoms* are the combination of your subjective feelings and the events that happen to your body. Back pain, vomiting, fatigue, and depression are all examples of symptoms (which can also be complaints).

Signs are the objective and verifiable marks of disease left on the body. You may not recognize these physical findings on your body, but your doctor is trained to notice them. For instance, the symptom of backache may be associated with the sign of muscle spasm. Vomiting may be associated with the signs of weight loss and dehydration. Other common signs include rashes, jaundice (yellow skin and eyes), or skin infection. You are usually aware of signs like these. However, other signs of disease are less obvious, such as an enlarged liver or spleen. By identifying the signs correctly, the doctor can arrive at the proper diagnosis. For example, the doctor may find an enlarged liver and jaundice as signs of hepatitis. Signs will provide your doctor with important clues as to how to proceed with the work-up and treatment plan.

THE CONSTELLATION OF FINDINGS

If you experience multiple symptoms and signs, it is known as a constellation of findings. Some of these signs and symptoms are more bothersome than others. It is important to let your doctor know what you are experiencing. It is particularly useful if you organize your complaints, symptoms, and signs in order of their importance or concern. This list (preferably written out) will guide your physician and help both of you to focus on the most serious symptoms and signs. That way he will know where to start to at least treat the most incapacitating symptoms first. This does not mean that your doctor will ignore the symptoms and signs at the bottom of your list. Nor does it mean that these symptoms and signs are not important. You still need to let your doctor know all that is wrong and let his training and experience determine what information can be discounted.

If treatment is not working or the diagnosis is in question, your doctor may revisit your list when considering alternative diagnoses and treatments. Sometimes the very sign that you or your doctor initially thought was insignificant may prove the key to unlocking the mystery of your illness. For example, a patient goes to the doctor complaining of a cough that won't go away and feeling tired. The doctor orders a chest x-ray, thinking the patient has pneumonia. However, the chest x-ray is negative—no pneumonia. Back to square one, so the doctor talks with the patient again. This time the patient mentions his swelling feet. The doctor then puts all of the symptoms and signs together to determine that the patient is suffering from heart disease. The doctor orders tests which indicate that heart disease is the correct diagnosis. It was only after revisiting the symptoms and signs that the doctor got the correct diagnosis.

Besides symptoms and signs, be sure to tell your physician about any special feelings or concerns that you may have regarding your illness. You should also notify him of any changes in habits or routines; such as, changes in your sleep, appetite, or bowel habits. It might be useful to also explain how the particular symptoms and signs are affecting your life and your family.

Exercise 8-1 provides one place for you to outline your signs and symptoms. Once you have completed it, bring a copy of it to your appointment. You can either give it to your doctor for review and inclusion in your medical records, or you can refer to it during the course of your appointment.

INSIDER'S HINT
....
Writing down your symptoms and signs commits you to being prepared.

KEEPING MEDICAL RECORDS

You are the sum total of your past. This includes your individual experience and your familial genetics. For some illnesses like diabetes, heart disease, and breast cancer, there is frequently a strong family history for individuals afflicted by these diseases.

When you go to the doctor, you will be asked many questions about your medical past. Some questions may be quite personal and potentially embarrassing. Other questions may require information that you would not normally have readily available. There are also those questions for which you may not want to admit the answers out loud.

Many people get a bit anxious or nervous around their doctor, especially if it is a first visit. It can be difficult to recall details about present and past health issues. To help keep track of and utilize your own personal and family medical history, we provide a form, Exercise 8-2. In the privacy of your own home you can research and answer questions without pressure or time constraints. This way, you'll never forget what strange disease Aunt Mazie had, and you will minimize the risk of forgetting important details for an appointment.

INSIDER'S HINT

Take the time to complete—then bring—a personal and family medical history to your appointment, particularly if it's your first visit with the doctor.

WHAT ARE ALL OF THESE PILL BOTTLES?

It is crucial that doctors have the correct information about a patient's medications. We recommend that for all medications you are currently taking, write down the following information:
- The name (generic or non-generic) of the medication.
- The quantity (dose) you are taking at one time.
- The number of times (frequency) you take it during the day, week, or month.
- How you are taking the medication, if it is different than the prescription.

Exercise 8-3 on page 112 will help you to organize this information. You should even keep this information in your wallet or purse. Should you ever end up in the ER, it will provide valuable information to the ER doctors. If it is difficult for you to write down this information because of poor mobility or vision, then seek out a friend, neighbor, or family member to assist you.

Another option is to bring all of your pill bottles to the appointment. Then the doctor can read directly from the bottles themselves and get the correct information into your medical records summary.

If some pill bottles have been misplaced, you should be able to enlist the help of your pharmacist, who can provide a comprehensive list of your medications. Of course, if you get your prescriptions filled at more than one pharmacy, you will need to contact those pharmacists too.

GATHERING ALL OF YOUR MEDICAL RECORDS

All in all, you will get the most out of a visit to a new doctor if she also gets the following medical records.
- Previous doctor's chart notes regarding diagnoses, physical findings, and treatment.
- Previous test results.
- Previous lab reports.
- Previous x-rays and imaging studies.

Not only does this provide your new doctor with all available information about your illness and health, but it allows her to contact your previous doctor for clarification of information. It also spares you the trouble, discomfort, and expense of repeating tests and procedures that have already been done.

To make sure your new doctor gets your medical records.
- Contact your referring/previous doctor and request copies of your chart, test results, lab reports, and x-rays.
- Give the previous doctor and his staff advance notice to copy and assemble your records.
- Pick up your records in person from your previous doctor's office. (You'll be asked to sign a release form.)
- Ask your new doctor if you need to drop off the medical records before your visit.
- Deliver your medical records with a cover letter (see Exercise 8-4 on page 113) to your new doctor.

Other materials and information that you may want to take with you include:
- Specific questions you want to ask the doctor during the appointment. Exercise 8-5 on page 114 provides a format for organizing your questions.
- Relevant magazine articles about your illness that you would like to discuss with your doctor.
- Information discovered on the Internet that you want to share with your doctor.

EMOTIONAL PREPARATION FOR THE APPOINTMENT

If you have followed all of the steps and done the exercises mentioned in this chapter to the best of your ability, then you are probably ready—at least on the outside. It is still normal to worry before a doctor's appointment. People often let their imaginations get the best of them during times of trouble, especially when they are anxious about their health.

One way to deal with worry is to make a list of your expectations and fears concerning your health and the outcome of the appointment. Once you have put them down on paper, think of two ways that you can overcome your fears and ensure that your expectations are met by you and your doctor. Exercise 8-6 on page 115 will guide you through this process. You might want to take a copy of this exercise with you to the doctor's appointment to make sure your expectations and fears are addressed by the end of your visit.

EXERCISE 8-1

Complaints, Symptoms, and Signs

1. Listing each complaint and symptom in order of importance, provide the following information:

COMPLAINT	DATE FIRST NOTICED	WAS ONSET SUDDEN OR SLOW	HOW OFTEN DOES IT OCCUR?

2. Describe your major health problem.

3. What have been the characteristics and course of your illness? Do you have any of the following signs? Circle appropriate responses.

a. Change in weight: Y   N   How much: _____

b. Change in appetite: Y   N   Increase or Decrease: _____

c. Change in sleep patterns: Y N Describe:_____

d. Fever: Y   N   Current temperature: _____

e. Chills: Y   N   For how long: _____

f. Night Sweats: Y   N   Describe:_____

g. Fatigue: Y   N   Describe:_____

h. Rash or Hives: Y   N   Describe:_____

Complaints, Symptoms, and Signs *(cont.)*

i. Cough: Y   N   Describe:_____

_____

j. Itch: Y   N   Describe:_____

_____

k. Diarrhea: Y   N   Describe:_____

_____

l. Jaundice: Y   N   Describe:_____

_____

m. Other: _____

_____

4. How have your complaints, symptoms, and signs affected you or your family?

_____

_____

_____

_____

_____

_____

_____

_____

_____

_____

Personal and Family Medical History Form

PERSONAL INFORMATION

Name: _____

DOB: _____ Age: ___ Birthplace: _____

Sex: _____ Marital Status: single   married   divorced

Race: _____

SOCIAL INFORMATION

Occupation: _____

Religion: _____

Highest Level of Completed Education: _____

List the countries you have traveled to: _____

_____

Have you served in the military: Y   N

Where: _____

_____

PAST MEDICAL HISTORY

Check which childhood diseases you have had:

___ chicken pox   ___ mumps

___ measles   ___ rubella

___ other, name: _____

Check which immunizations you have had:

___ diphtheria   ___ hepatitis A, date: _____

___ tetanus, date: _____   ___ hepatitis B

___ pertussis   ___ pneumococcal

___ combined DTP/DT   ___ influenza, date: _____

___ polio   ___ TB skin test, date: _____

___ measles, mumps, rubella   ___ other: _____

EXERCISE 8-2

Personal and Family Medical History Form

(cont.)

PAST MEDICAL HISTORY

List your adult diseases (such as pneumonia or diabetes):

_____   _____

_____   _____

_____   _____

List all of your broken bones, if applicable:

_____   _____

_____   _____

_____   _____

Check which traumas you have you suffered from:

____ third degree burns, what part of your body:_____

____ gunshot wound, what part of your body: _____

____ traumatic injuries, what were they: _____

____ unconsciousness as a result of an injury

____ poisonings, what was the poison:_____

What is your blood type: _____

Have you had any blood transfusions: Y   N

When:_____

List all of your past operations:

_____   _____

_____   _____

_____   _____

_____   _____

List all of your past hospitalizations:

_____   _____

_____   _____

_____   _____

EXERCISE 8-2

Personal and Family Medical History Form
(cont.)
PAST MEDICAL HISTORY (CONT.)

List all medications you are currently taking:

_____   _____

_____   _____

_____   _____

Have you ever experienced an allergy or side effect
to a medication: Y   N

Name the drug: _____

Reaction: _____

List all of your allergies:

_____   _____

_____   _____

_____   _____

Have you been treated for a psychiatric illness: Y   N

List your illness: _____

When were you treated: _____

LIFESTYLE QUESTIONS:

Do you exercise?:   ___no   ___occasionally   ___regularly

Do you follow a special diet?:   Y   N

Describe it: _____

_____

_____

Personal and Family Medical History Form
(cont.)

PAST MEDICAL HISTORY (CONT.)

Do you drink coffee, tea or caffeinated sodas?: Y   N

How often: _____

Do you drink alcoholic beverages?   Y   N

How often: _____

What type of alcohol do you drink:

Have you ever been advised to decrease or stop
your alcohol consumption?   Y   N

When: _____

Have you ever used illicit drugs?   Y   N

Do you or did you ever smoke?   Y   N

How many packs per day _____   For how many years _____

Do you chew tobacco?   Y   N

How many tins per day _____   For how many years _____

Do you take vitamin tablets?   Y   N

What kind: _____

Are you sexually active?:   Y   N

FAMILY MEDICAL HISTORY

Check if your parents or other blood relatives have had any of the
following diseases:

____ arthritis	____ alzheimer's
____ breast cancer	____ colon cancer
____ lung cancer	____ skin cancer
____ ovarian cancer	____ cataracts
____ diabetes	____ glaucoma
____ heart disease	____ osteoporosis
____ strokes	____ thyroid disorders
____ colitis	____ neurological disease (MS, ALS)
____ high blood pressure	____ psoriasis
____ high cholesterol	____ peptic ulcer disease

FOR WOMEN:

What was the start date of your last period: _____

How long does your cycle last: _____

Have you ever been pregnant: Y N

How many times_____

Have you ever had an abortion: Y N

Have you ever had a miscarriage: Y N

EXERCISE 8-3

Medication Information Form

List below the name, dose, and frequency of the medication that you are currently taking. Include both prescription and over-the-counter medications.

Medication	Dose	Frequency

Do you have any allergies or side effects to medications?   Y N

If yes, what kind of side effects do you have and to which medications:

1.

2.

3.

4.

EXERCISE 8-4

Chart Cover Letter

Patient Name: _____ Date of Birth: _____

Address: _____

Work Number: _____ Home Number: _____

Primary Care Physician: _____

Insurance: _____

Physician Referring You to This Doctor: _____

Summarize Reason For Seeing This Doctor: _____

_____

_____

_____

_____

_____

_____

_____

_____

_____

_____

_____

_____

_____

_____

_____

_____

_____

_____

_____

_____

_____

_____

_____

_____

_____

_____

Questions to Ask Your Doctor

In the following space, write out any questions that you want to ask your doctor during your appointment. Take this sheet with you to your appointment. You can then write down the doctor's answer next to your question. This sheet can then be incorporated into your personal medical records for future reference.

1. Question: _____

   _____

   Answer: _____

   _____

   _____

2. Question: _____

   _____

   Answer: _____

   _____

   _____

3. Question: _____

   _____

   Answer: _____

   _____

   _____

4. Question: _____

   _____

   Answer: _____

   _____

   _____

5. Question: _____

   _____

   Answer: _____

   _____

   _____

Expectations and Fears

1. List your expectations concerning your health status and your doctor's appointment:

_____   _____

_____   _____

_____   _____

_____   _____

2. What can you do, think, feel or say in order to better meet and accomplish your expectations?

_____

_____

_____

_____

3. List your fears concerning your health status and your doctor's appointment:

_____   _____

_____   _____

_____   _____

4. What can you do, think, feel, or say in order to overcome or at least lessen your fears:

_____

_____

_____

_____

_____

_____

_____

_____

Chapter 9

The Appointment

Peter Gardner awoke at 4 A.M. Monday morning feeling like his right foot was on fire. By 9 A.M. he was unable to walk due to the pain. His wife called her doctor and got an appointment for him later that morning. Mr. Gardner limped into the office using his trusty 3-iron for a cane. Dr. Baker took a quick history and performed a quick exam. The doctor told Mr. Gardner that she would need to take a little fluid out of his big toe joint and analyze it in her office lab. Mr. Gardner assumed that this couldn't hurt any more than he was already hurting, so he said "OK." Was he ever wrong! The needle felt like a hot dagger driven into the bone.

By the time Dr. Baker returned from her office lab, Mr. Gardner's stomach was queasy and his foot hurt like hell. Mr. Gardner had gout, she said, and would need to take some pills. Mr. Gardner listened but didn't really hear her because he was so overwhelmed by the pain. The only thing on his mind was getting home and back to bed.

Two weeks later, Mr. Gardner was back to golfing and had no pain in his big toe. Since he felt fine, he wasn't sure why he should go back for his follow-up appointment with Dr. Baker. All he could remember was the pain that the doctor had inflicted upon him. He was concerned about his original joint pain episode, but preferred to ignore the whole issue hoping that it would never reappear. Mrs. Gardner, on the other hand, was worried that if the gout (a type of arthritis) became persistent she would end up having to push her husband around in a wheelchair for the rest of his life. She insisted on the follow-up visit and even went along to make sure that she also under-stood his problem.

During the appointment, Dr. Baker sensed that Mr. Gardner had not learned much from the previous appointment. She took extra time explaining the results of the lab tests. Then she gave them a brochure about gout, which outlined how to avoid another attack with preventive measures such as watching his diet, not drinking too much alcohol, and taking a daily medication. As they left the office, Mr. Gardner thanked his wife for insisting on the follow-up visit. He felt that his time was well spent. Mrs. Gardner just smiled.

BEFORE THE APPOINTMENT

CHECK YOUR FRAME OF MIND. Feeling angry or frustrated because the last 16 doctors you saw could not diagnose or treat your problem? That doesn't mean your new doctor won't be able to treat you. Being angry right from the start will put your new doctor on the defensive. It's human nature. Consider this first appointment with this new doctor as a fresh start on a new treatment journey.

INSIDER'S HINT

It helps to give doctors a reason to go that extra mile for you.

PREPARE FOR A WAIT, BRING YOUR WHITTLIN'. Remember to bring something constructive to do, such as needlepoint, your portable computer, or a book to read because your doctor might be running late. All sorts of forces conspire to make a physician late. Unexpected minor and major emergencies with other patients could send your doctor to the hospital. An emergency "squeeze-in," phone calls from other doctors, and lab results all might cause doctors to get behind schedule.

CALL YOUR DOCTOR IF YOU ARE RUNNING LATE. We all know that unexpected circumstances occur, and being late is sometimes unavoidable. If you are running behind schedule, let your doctor's office know. Many offices will not be able to see you if you are over 15 to 30 minutes late unless you have called ahead. If you don't let the office know you're running late, your absence may be noted as a "no show." If this hap-pens repeatedly, many offices will no longer see you. By calling to let them know you will be late, the doctor's staff might be able to fit you in when you arrive or at least let you know that you need to resched-ule the appointment for another time.

ARRIVE EARLY TO COMPLETE THE FORMS. If this is your initial visit with this doctor, you will often be asked to arrive early to fill out forms. You will want to give the receptionist copies of the materials you gathered or completed in preparation for the visit (see Chapter 8). The doctor may like to review these materials before meeting you in the exam room.

GETTING THE MOST OUT OF YOUR TIME

In this day and age, everyone is busy. Unfortunately, a doctor's time is even more limited than most. The length of an office visit depends on the expected complexity of your problems. A new patient office visit may be anywhere from 30 to 60 minutes. Return visits are usually between 10 and 30 minutes. Good doctors are popular doctors and thus are busy with many patients. Doctors who are employees of an HMO or other managed care organization even may be told how much time is permissible with each patient.

If even modest delays occur, it can have repercussions throughout the rest of the day. Subsequent patients may have to wait or get less time with the doctor. Therefore, we recommend that you optimize your time spent with your doctor.

Organization and preparation are two ways to maximize the use of your time during the appointment. Another is prioritization. If you have seven problems you would like to discuss and only have 15 to 30 minutes, it is unlikely that anything will be addressed in an adequate fashion if all seven are brought up. Go ahead and mention all of your concerns, but try to focus on the chief complaint. Present the one or two issues of major importance and perhaps save the others for another visit once the bigger problems are under treatment.

To help you utilize your office visit time effectively, try to divide the visit into its smaller components. This is not meant as a rigid protocol to be timed with a stopwatch! This is simply a guide. For a typical 30-minute first visit and a 15-minute follow-up visit you may wish to divide your appointment as follows:

VISIT COMPONENT	FIRST APPOINTMENT		FOLLOW-UP APPOINTMENT	
	MINUTES	%	MINUTES	%
Greeting	2	6	1	7
Symptom Reporting	5	17	2	13
Physical Exam	5	17	1	7
Diagnosis	6	20	1	7
Treatment	6	20	5	33
Patient's Other Needs	2	7	1	7
Questions	3	10	3	19
Summary or future plans	1	3	1	7
	30	100	15	100

Looking at the office visit in this manner, you can understand why a large number of issues, illnesses, diagnoses, and concerns cannot be dealt with at a single visit.

- Focus primarily on the primary problem.
- Spend the remainder of the time on secondary problems.
- If needed, make an additional appointment in order to fully understand your problem, its ramifications, and treatment options.
- If needed, make an additional appointment to discuss secondary problems.

Becoming informed and proactive in your health care is not always quick or easy. Exercise 9-1 will help you to organize your time.

THE FIRST APPOINTMENT

LEARNING ABOUT YOUR CHIEF COMPLAINT AND SYMPTOMS Following introductions and greetings, the doctor will proceed with asking you about your chief complaint, or problems you are experiencing (Chapter 8). In medical school, doctors are taught to follow the SOAP approach (Chapter 1) to obtain all the needed information from you in an efficient manner. However, how your story is obtained depends upon the doctor's style and on how concisely you present it. Some physicians will let you tell your story without interrupting you, and then ask questions at the end. Others will constantly interrupt. Whichever your doctor's style, try to be sure the doctor gets your whole story to your satisfaction. You don't want to leave the appointment thinking your doctor didn't fully understand your problem. Exercise 8-1 on page 105 will help you convey your medical complaints and answer questions.

DISCOVERING YOUR MEDICAL HISTORY. After discussing the details of your chief complaint, the doctor will review your medical history. (The information in exercises 8-2, 8-3, and 8-6 as well as other records that you brought with you will be valuable is assessing your medical history.) Upon reviewing all of the information, the doctor may wish to ask more questions to obtain other detailed information or to clarify any inconsistencies for accuracy.

PERFORMING THE PHYSICAL EXAM. The next part of the appointment is "the laying on of the hands" by the doctor. The physical exam should be done in a gentle and respectful manner. However, you should still be prepared to experience some discomfort, maybe outright pain, and perhaps embarrassment. Talking to your doctor throughout the exam may put you more at ease and help you deal with the discomfort, pain, or embarrassment.

FEEL FREE TO TALK OR ASK QUESTIONS DURING THE PHYSICAL EXAM. You will not only learn more about your body and how to evaluate it, but you will also learn about how your doctor practices medicine. (Though there are times when it will be necessary to be silent such as when she uses a stethoscope and listens to your heart and lungs.) Most importantly, you will learn how your doctor handles questions by a curious, actively involved patient. This knowledge will be useful later on when you need to ask possibly more difficult questions about your diagnosis and treatment.

Finally, besides observing your symptoms and signs, the doctor should also take some time during the appointment to get to know you, the patient. By doing so, the doctor will be better able to understand you and your needs in relation to your illness.

WHAT'S PROPER, WHAT'S NOT? Being poked, prodded, inspected, and scoped in various stages of undress, there are certain norms as to what is considered proper and what is not. You should be allowed to disrobe in privacy and given a gown, either cloth or paper, for warmth and modesty. It is always proper to have your body covered when you are just talking to the doctor. During an exam, it is proper to expose only the area of the body that is being examined at that time. All other parts or areas not being examined should be covered or draped.

If you wish, it is proper to ask to have a nurse present for your exam. Pelvic exams should be observed by a female nurse. In some cases, a nurse may be present even during exams where the doctor and patient are of the same gender. Physicians may do breast and male genital and rectal exams without another person present, but again only if you are comfortable with this. Children should be examined with their parents or legal guardian present, unless it is a medical emergency. If you have any specific fears or concerns, ask about them before the exam so that they can be addressed to your satisfaction. It is a doctor's goal to make you feel as comfortable as possible during the examination.

CAN YOU GET AN INITIAL DIAGNOSIS? After the first visit, the doctor should have an inkling as to whether something is wrong with you and tell you her preliminary concerns. She should be able to give you a preliminary assessment and a *differential diagnosis*. A differential diagnosis is a listing of the most likely possibilities that explain your symptoms and physical findings. Sometimes, this diagnosis may be broadly defined and at best left vague, such as "infection" or "back pain." At other times, the differential diagnosis may be more specific, for example, the infection is caused by acute sinusitis or pneumonia; or back pain is due to a herniated disc or muscle injury. With luck, after the first visit, the doctor may even know what is precisely wrong with you. However, if she doesn't, she may formulate a *working diagnosis*. A working diagnosis is a temporary opinion from which the doctor will base further evaluation and the initial treatment. This diagnosis will evolve over time and hopefully become more precise. See Chapter 11 for a more detailed discussion about diagnosis.

CAN YOU GET A PRELIMINARY TREATMENT PLAN? On the basis of your differential or working diagnosis, your doctor may formulate a preliminary treatment plan. This might be simple observation over time to see what develops, or you may start on a therapeutic trial with medication. Doctors will often treat your symptoms while trying to determine specifically what disease to treat. When your disease is finally diagnosed then you should expect the doctor to focus your treatment plan on curing or slowing down the disease and not just treating the symptoms. See Chapter 12 for a more detailed discussion on treatment.

"THIS MIGHT BE A STUPID QUESTION, BUT…" There is no such thing as a stupid question. If you have lingering questions that are nagging you, just ask them. It is better to ask a question and receive an answer that will satisfy a worry or concern, then to leave the appointment and fret about the unknown. If the doctor is a skilled communicator, you'll never even know if you did ask a dumb question. Besides, your doctor does not expect you to be an expert in medical matters, so it is normal for a patient to ask both basic and complicated questions. Sometimes the doctor may appear to be pressed for time and in a hurry to get on to the next appointment. If it becomes clear that there isn't enough time to get all of your questions answered, tell the doctor that you want a follow-up appointment to finish your discussion.

EXPECT THE UNEXPECTED! Allow time in your schedule to accommodate lab tests or minor procedures that may need to be performed after the appointment. Give yourself at least an hour until your next scheduled appointment or meeting.

Establish a contingency plan for the possibility of not being able to go home on time. Emergency hospital admission straight from the doctor's office is uncommon, but it still does occur.

FIND OUT HOW TO GET INFORMATION AFTER THE APPOINTMENT. Every doctor's office has its own policy about how to convey information to you. Some offices will send you a written note outlining the test results. Other practices might have a nurse call and explain the results to you over the telephone. Then again, you might be asked to return for another visit to discuss your test results and how they impact your health and treatment plan. Just make sure you understand your doctor's policy and practices before leaving the exam room.

THE FOLLOW-UP APPOINTMENT

The follow-up visit allows you and your doctor to examine your progress and adjust your treatment plan. It provides an opportunity for ensuring that you are receiving adequate care.

HOW OFTEN DO YOU NEED TO GO FOR FOLLOW-UP CARE? Follow-up visits can range from every several days to only on a semi-annual or annual basis. Typically, your doctor will schedule your first follow-up appointment for two to four weeks after the first appointment. Then depending upon the severity of your illness and the complexity level of your treatment, you may need to be seen more or less frequently. As you might expect, if your progress is not good, then you will be seen more frequently. If you are doing well, then you may be seen less frequently.

If your doctor asks to see you on a basis that is more or less frequent than you think is appropriate, ask for an explanation or an earlier appointment. However, for the sake of your time and money, you should make certain that more visits are necessary. Mr. Gardner, in the opening story, wasn't even sure he needed a follow-up appointment. His symptoms had resolved, but he was worried that he could suffer another arthritis attack. His follow-up appointment helped him to better understand his diagnosis of gout and the principles of its management. Mr. Gardner should now only need one to two follow-up visits a year to assure control of his disease.

WHAT HAPPENS DURING A FOLLOW-UP EXAM? Follow-up visits provide you the opportunity to review your progress with your doctor. Your doctor will ask you about your symptoms and also determine if the prescribed therapy is working. The doctor will review any new information to see if the working diagnosis still fits, especially in light of any new symptoms or signs that you might have developed since your last visit.

At each revisit, you will discuss the results of any previously ordered tests and how they relate to your diagnosis. Do the results support or refute the working diagnosis? The test results may also alter your treatment plan and suggest a new direction. During the follow-up, the doctor will also review your medications. He will determine if you are taking them correctly and will be looking for information on possible side effects. Side effects may outweigh the benefits of your treatment and necessitate changes in your medications and treatment.

The follow-up appointment will be more valuable if you come prepared with accurate information and a set of questions. We recommend keeping an ongoing **MEDICAL LOG** to track health events over the course of your illness. Exercise 9-2 illustrates how to develop this medical log, which should, at the least, contain information on the date of a health event or activity; the time of day (if significant); the symptoms, objective signs, and any important changes in them; your important feelings and observations; and short summaries of all medical office visits or diagnostic testing. Exercise 9-3 on page 130 will help you to organize your thoughts and questions.

It is not necessary, nor is it recommended, that you recite your medical log, word for word, at your follow-up appointment. If your health problems have been complicated, and your medical log is extensive, bring a summary of the medical log to the appointment. Exercise 9-4 shows how you could format this summary.

ARE YOU STILL WILLING TO FOLLOW-THROUGH WITH THE TREATMENT PLAN? This important question should be discussed at a follow-up appointment. You are the one primarily responsible for your getting well. The best doctor with the best plan and the best bedside manner cannot help anyone if they do not cooperate. As part of the follow-up appointment, you should discuss with your doctor whether or not you still agree with and can follow through with the treatment plan. Health professionals call this compliance, which means following the prescribed instructions.

If you believe that your working diagnosis is correct and your treatment plan is good, then following it should be easy, especially if you are seeing some progress. However, there may be times when you have good intentions but for practical purposes you just can't seem to devote time on a daily basis to your treatment. If you face this dilemma, talk to your doctor and explore other treatment or medication options that would work better for you. It is better to take part in a less ambitious but more realistic treatment plan, than to attempt to follow a plan that looks and sounds great but is unrealistic; one with which you cannot possibly follow.

Mr. Gardner, from this chapter's introductory story, faithfully took his medication every day after learning about his gout. Still, neither he nor Dr. Baker understood why he continued to have periodic gout attacks. That is, until Mr. Gardner told her that he still stopped off at a tavern on paydays with the guys from work to relax and enjoy a few beers. In this instance, Mr. Gardner was only following part of his treatment plan.

LIVING BETWEEN VISITS
Many people look to their doctor and his staff for support and comfort during the treatment process, especially early in the course of a severe illness. Looking for hope, patients cling to the words of their doctor, just trying to survive the days between office visits. This is especially true with strong and nurturing caregivers

If you find yourself relying too much on your doctor, it is imperative that you find alternative sources of support. Your family, friends, church, and support groups are good options. These groups or individuals may be better equipped to provide you with the daily comfort, love, friendship, and support you need. They also will most likely have more time available to meet many of your special needs. Think of your doctor as a touchstone. She is there to guide and comfort you when you require professional advice, medical direction, and assurance that cannot be achieved elsewhere. Dr. Bernie Siegel has written an excellent book on the topic called, *How to Live Between Office Visits.*

SHOULD YOU CALL AFTER HOURS?

Doctor's offices have set hours like any other business. In the best of circumstances, most problems would be dealt with during the course of a normal day. But when they can't, your doctor, or his covering physician, should be available to you 24 hours a day, 7 days a week.

A doctor's 24-hour availability has been one of the traditional foundations of medical practice. It should not be misused or abused and should be reserved only for what is thought to be an urgent situation. Calling for problems that are chronic and without change should also be avoided. It is unnecessary and thoughtless to call a doctor at 3 A.M. for cold symptoms or an itch that has been present for the last two weeks.

The following recommendations will help you get the care you need after hours.

PREPARE THE CALL. Write down your symptoms and signs. Also write down a list of the current medications you are taking.

FIND OUT IF YOUR PHARMACY IS OPEN. If not, find one that is open. Have the pharmacy's phone number available to give to your doctor, so he will be able to call in a prescription, if needed.

CALL YOUR DOCTOR'S OFFICE NUMBER. It will ring through to the answering service. You will have to wait for the doctor to call you back, so provide a telephone number where you can be reached.

DESCRIBE YOUR PROBLEMS TO THE DOCTOR CLEARLY AND CONCISELY TO ENSURE A BETTER EVALUATION OVER THE TELEPHONE. After hours, the greatest problem for both patient and physician is making decisions based upon a telephone conversation. Without the benefit of a physical exam, chart, or diagnostic test, there are inherent limitations to a doctor's evaluation. This is especially true if the call is handled by the covering doctor, who isn't familiar with a particular patient. This is why preparation before calling is important.

BE PREPARED TO GO TO THE EMERGENCY ROOM. If the symptoms seem serious, the answering doctor may ask that you be evaluated in an ER either by himself or the ER staff.

CALL BACK AND SEEK FURTHER ADVISE, IF NEEDED. It is your responsibility to call back and seek further advice, if your condition worsens following the telephone consultation.

CALL 911 IF YOU CAN'T WAIT FOR THE DOCTOR TO CALL YOU. If you think your problem is life-threatening, do not waste time. Call 911 immediately.

The response to an after-hours call may not provide you with all the answers and services you want. Hopefully, though, it will provide you with what you need at that time.

THE APPOINTMENT REVIEW

When you see a doctor, especially a new one, family and friends are bound to ask about the appointment. "Did you like your doctor?" "Did they find out what is wrong?" "What can you do about it?" The best time to review your impressions of the visit and the doctor is right after the visit. Talk with family and friends to help you understand what you learned during the appointment. You might even want to write your impressions in your medical log.

Even if you have settled into a longer-term relationship with your doctor, it is important to reevaluate that relationship. Has your doctor met most of your goals, needs, and expectations? Have your questions and concerns been addressed thoroughly and compassionately? If you are having serious second thoughts about your physician, then it may be time to consider seeing someone else.

EXERCISE 9-1

Time Management of Your Appointment

Before your visit, find out from your doctor's office about how much time will be scheduled for your appointment. Use the following breakdown to budget the amount of time you would like to see spent on each area. During your visit, if you feel that the time is not being spent appropriately, refer to this exercise to help get back on course.

Stage of the Visit	Minutes
Greeting*	_____
Symptom Reporting*	_____
Patient's Needs*	_____
Diagnosis	_____
Treatment	_____
Physical Exam	_____
Questions	_____
Summary or Future Plans	_____
Total Time	_____

---

*It is during these components of the visit that you can go through your HOPE format developed in Exercise 1-1.

EXERCISE 9-2

Medical Logs

These logs are examples for starting your own medical logs. These should be kept with your personal medical records. Enlarge this record to 200% on a copier.

SYMPTOMS LOG

Date & Time	Symptoms	Objective Signs	Changes Since Onset	Feelings/ Observations

OFFICE VISIT AND TELEPHONE LOG

Date	Name	Location of Visit	Summary of Phone Conv.	Summary of Office Visit	Tests or Procedures Performed	Results

EXERCISE 9-3

Revisit Questions

Here are some questions to ask your doctor during your revisit.

DIAGNOSTIC AND TREATMENT QUESTIONS

1. Have I been willing to follow through on my treatment plan?

Y   N

2. Is the treatment/medication working?   Y   N

3. Am I better or worse?   Y   N

4. Do I need to have any additional tests?

If yes, what are they?   Y   N

_____

_____

_____

5. Do I have any complications from the treatment
or side effects from the medications?   Y   N

_____

_____

_____

6. Am I taking my medicine in the manner that you prescribed?

Y   N

7. Will I have to make any changes to my treatment plan?
If yes, what are they?   Y   N

_____

_____

_____

(Share with your doctor any articles you have read that deal with your illness. Ask for his opinion about them and if the information is applicable to your illness.)

EXERCISE 9-3

Revisit Questions *(cont.)*

EMOTIONAL SUPPORT QUESTIONS

1. I would like to express my worries and concerns. They are:

_____

_____

_____

2. This may seem like a simple question, but:

_____

_____

_____

3. I am embarrassed to ask, but:

_____

_____

_____

4. Can you recommend a support group? Or reading material?

_____

_____

EXERCISE 9-4

Medical Log Summary Sheet

1. List any new signs or symptoms you have experienced since your last visit. For each sign and symptom, briefly describe it and state when you first became aware of it. List them in order of decreasing severity (most severe first).

Signs/Symptoms	Onset Date
_____	_____
_____	_____
_____	_____
_____	_____
_____	_____
_____	_____
_____	_____
_____	_____
_____	_____
_____	_____
_____	_____

2. How are you currently feeling?

_____

_____

_____

3. What can you say about what has changed for you since your last visit?

_____

_____

_____

4. Indicate any problems you have encountered while following your treatment.

_____

_____

Chapter 10

The Work-Up

Tom was working at the shipyard as he had done on countless days in the past. He was usually careful about lifting, but on this particular day he was in a hurry and lifted a box in haste. Suddenly, he felt an exquisite zap of pain radiating down his right leg. He tried to ignore it, hoping it would vanish as quickly as it came, but as the day went on, the pain only worsened. By quitting time his back was in spasm, he was no longer able to work and even had trouble standing.

Tom went to see his doctor the very next day. Dr. Martin prescribed bed rest, pain medications, and muscle relaxants. After two weeks Tom had not improved. In fact, he was worse; now his whole leg felt totally numb and his foot was beginning to feel weak. Dr. Martin believed that Tom had a herniated disk, which was beginning to cause nerve damage. The doctor also thought that a test was needed to confirm his diagnosis and to help plan further therapy.

Without asking, Tom assumed he would have to have a painful myelogram, an exam that looks at the spinal nerve roots and discs. He knew about the test because his father had one some years past to evaluate similar symptoms. Tom remembered his father's vivid description of being strapped onto a table and experiencing severe pain as a thick oily substance was injected into his spine with a large needle. Tom recalled the severe headache that his dad suffered immediately after the test and the chronic headaches he had for months afterwards. To this day his father has never completely recovered. In fact, his dad has continuing back pain due to scarred nerves caused by the procedure.

Tom wanted no part of this test. He would rather live with the pain than to submit to this form of controlled torture. Dr. Martin, however, reassured him that things are different today and that myelograms are rarely performed. The doctor told Tom that they would do an MRI scan (magnetic resonance imaging) instead. Tom would just have to sit in a relatively enclosed space where he could listen to some music, and perhaps even fall asleep, while the test is performed. No needles, no straps, and no pain. And if Tom felt claustrophobic, Dr. Martin assured Tom he would be given a mild sedative to make him feel more comfortable.

Somewhat skeptical, Tom went for his MRI. To his surprise, the test was just as it was described. Two days later, Dr. Martin called and gave Tom the details of his diagnosis along with some treatment options.

TESTING ... ONE, TWO, THREE

Modern medicine has evolved dramatically in the area of diagnostic testing. A woman no longer needs to "wait for the rabbit to die" in order to find out that she is pregnant. Instead, in the privacy of her own home, she can do an accurate home pregnancy test bought off the supermarket shelf. Not only has diagnostic testing progressed to allow in-home testing, but tests that were previously only done in the hospital can now be done in the doctor's office on an outpatient basis.

Additionally, an unparalleled array of sophisticated and reliable testing is now available to take the element of uncertainty out of many diagnoses. Diseases that once required surgery to be diagnosed can now be diagnosed with computer generated imaging and biopsy guided techniques. Today, tests are safer, quicker, less expensive, more reliable, and require less preparation and recovery time.

THE CATEGORIES OF TESTING

If your diagnosis is not known with certainty at the end of your visit, the doctor will want to perform a workup. A workup is a series of tests done in order to rule in or out (prove or disprove) the various possibilities in your differential diagnosis.

The tests your doctor orders can be broken down into routine, specialized, and esoteric or experimental.

ROUTINE TESTS. These are the tests performed most frequently by doctors. Their purpose is to screen for diseases; to diagnose frequently occurring problems, such as urinary tract infections, diabetes, thyroid disease, and anemia; to detect side effects of medications, such as hypokalemia (low potassium) in patients taking diuretics (water pill); to monitor your vital statistics such as height, weight, temperature, cholesterol, and blood pressure. Routine tests include blood tests, urinalysis, chest x-rays, and mammograms.

SPECIALIZED TESTS. These tests are still commonly performed by doctors, but not ordered routinely. They are performed to confirm a specific diagnosis or to answer a specific question. Specialized tests include imaging exams, such as MRI scans to look for herniated disks or ultrasounds to look for kidney stones or gallstones.

ESOTERIC AND EXPERIMENTAL TESTS. These two types may or may not be mutually exclusive. Esoteric tests are uncommon tests. They may only be performed in a few laboratories around the country. Experimental tests, on the other hand, have not been firmly established by the medical community as being useful or valid; thus they often are not covered by insurance policies. Rare diseases or common diseases that strike in rare ways can be very difficult to detect and may require an esoteric or experimental test.

Esoteric tests include PET scans (positron emission tomography) and rare blood tests, and experimental tests include new research markers for genetic diseases.

THE THOUGHT-PROCESS BEHIND ORDERING TESTS

Two basic approaches are used to order tests. We call them "duck hunting" and sequential testing. Most doctors use a combination of both to outline a process for your work-up.

"DUCK HUNTING" APPROACH. Here, the doctor orders many tests at once hoping to arrive at a diagnosis quickly. He is primarily aiming in the general direction of a symptom, hoping the tests reveal something. "Duck hunting" is usually more expedient than sequential testing, but it is also more costly as unnecessary tests might be performed. There are merits to "duck hunting," but it is usually limited to illnesses that are difficult to diagnose or may require rapid treatment.

SEQUENTIAL TESTING APPROACH. Sequential testing is the most common work-up strategy, especially if the illness does not appear to be imminently life threatening. Under this approach, the doctor starts with your symptoms and signs and determines which tests will be done first. These tests are called *screening tests.* Usually those tests with the highest probability of confirming your diagnosis are performed first. Based upon the results of the screening tests, the doctor can then determine which tests should be ordered next. This sequential process continues until the doctor arrives at a diagnosis.

In the patient who complains of chest pain, for example, differential diagnoses could include angina pectoris, asthma, hiatal hernia with reflux esophagitis, chostochondritis, and pleurisy. Because angina is the most serious disorder and could lead to a myocardial infarction (heart attack) and even death, an electrocardiogram (EKG) would be the initial screening test. If abnormal, a more rapid investigation would ensue. If normal, a stress test would be the next logical step to see if the symptoms could be reproduced by stressing the heart with exercise. If the stress test is equivocal (ambiguous) or positive, an angiogram would be ordered to see whether medical, surgical, or even no therapy would be appropriate. If all of these tests point away from heart disease, then the doctor may proceed to investigate the possibility of lung, esophagus, or stomach diseases. Ordering lung, gastrointestinal (GI), and heart tests all at once would be exhausting, time consuming, expensive, and wasteful. Sequential testing provides for a logical approach that leads to a series of possible tests that have the best chance of uncovering a diagnosis. Sequential testing also helps to minimize the cost and the waste of medical resources.

UNDERSTANDING, AGREEMENT, AND INFORMED CONSENT

It's important that you understand the "why" of any tests—the logic behind a given test and the sequence in which the tests will be done. Understanding "why" it will be done and what will be done allows you to see how the test will benefit you directly. This also helps to alleviate any fears you may have about undergoing certain tests. If your doctor has not given you an explanation of your ordered tests, then you should ask for one prior to having them done. The explanation should include:
  • why the test is being ordered
  • who will administer the test

- where and when will the test take place
- what are the test's advantages and disadvantages
- what are the test's benefits and risks
- when will you get the test results

Not only is it your right to understand your work-up, but you should also agree with it. A doctor cannot perform a test on you without your consent. If you do object to what your doctor is ordering or don't understand, you need to tell your doctor right away. Perhaps he will realize that he hasn't adequately explained the tests to you. Or maybe you haven't conveyed to him your fears or religious and ethical concerns regarding certain tests. If your doctor knows this, then he can help you make a more informed decision about which tests would be best for you. You and your doctor can then discuss your test options and find some middle ground that offers the best compromise. The final say, however, is always yours.

For legal purposes you may be asked to sign a consent form. This documents the fact that the doctor has explained to you the procedure and its risks and benefits. By signing this form the patient legally consents to the test and assumes the risks of a properly performed procedure. Even after you have signed a consent form you can change your mind before the test is performed and ask that the consent form be returned or destroyed. Once the test is performed the consent form becomes a legal document. If a complication should occur it is the consent form that will be vital to documenting for both the patient and the doctor that appropriate procedures were followed. Exercise 10-1 will help you to organize the needed information for your tests. The governing and safety of experimental testing is discussed in Chapter 19.

OUTPATIENT TESTING

Unless your condition is serious or potentially serious, you probably do not need to be admitted to a hospital for testing. Most tests today are done almost exclusively on an outpatient basis. Typically, the procedure is done early in the day and the patient is allowed to go home after a certain amount of observation to ensure there are no complications.

An extremely common exception is if your doctor suspects a myocardial infarction (heart attack), because the most serious complications of heart attacks often occur in the first 24 to 72 hours. In this instance, you would probably be admitted to the hospital for serial testing of heart enzymes which usually takes 24 hours. If the heart attack diagnosis is ruled out, you can usually go home the next day.

ORGANIZING TESTS MORE EFFICIENTLY

Routine blood tests and x-rays are almost always available at a doctor's office. These tests can usually be done following your appointment without scheduling or a significant waiting time. However, if fasting blood work is required and you have not fasted on the day of your appointment, then you will need to return early one morning for the requisite testing.

Many times, tests need to be scheduled in different departments of the hospital or at a local laboratory. This creates special problems when you are trying to do the tests in a more efficient manner and sequence. If several tests are ordered, and are not needed on an urgent or semi-urgent basis, you should be able to have them scheduled at your convenience. You may be able to have them all scheduled for the same morning or afternoon.

In the unusual circumstance that one test would interfere with the performance of another, the physician will order tests in a particular sequence that may be less convenient to you. For example, residual barium following a barium enema would interfere with other x-ray studies of the abdomen for two to four days. Unless the barium enema is the most vital test, it probably should be performed last.

We recommend working with the nurse in your doctor's office. He or she can help you schedule your tests to more efficiently organize your work-up.

PREPARATION TIPS FOR TESTS Each test has different levels of preparation. Tests may require:
- no preparation at all
- overnight fasting (cholesterol checks, for example)
- consumption of fluids (for ultrasounds)
- sleep avoidance (for some EEG [electroencephalogram] tests)
- self administration of an enema (for a barium enema)
- special medications prior to the test

Ask about any required preparation and for any written instruction sheets for your tests. The written instructions help ensure proper preparation. If you're not properly prepared, you may have to reschedule the test in order to get valid results.

Ask for written instruction sheets for your tests.

ARE THE TESTS PAINFUL?

Even a simple blood test involves a needle stick and a little discomfort. Other tests, such as electrodiagnostic nerve testing (NCV, EMG), may be uncomfortable for some people and outright torture for others. How painful the test is often depends on two factors:

1. If you are generally more sensitive to pain and discomfort than most people you know, then any test might be more painful to you.
2. The skill of the individual who performs the test may make it more or less painful.

Ask your physician what pain if any to expect from a test. And make sure to let the doctor know what you experienced for future reference.

Some tests may be psychologically painful. An MRI places a person into a confining space in which he or she must lie perfectly still for what can amount to a lengthy period of time. If in your past, particularly your childhood, you had a bad experience with being held down or trapped in a small space, you might not be able to deal with the MRI scan.

It is best to discuss with your doctor any anxiety before you undergo the test. For some tests, you may need a mild sedative. Sometimes, though, even medication may not help. Even so, other tests might be available to evaluate your problem without putting you in a situation that causes mental anguish. Just ask your doctor.

ARE THE TESTS NECESSARY OR IS YOUR DOCTOR COVERING HER LEGAL BEHIND?

Over the past two decades, most doctors have changed their practice habits to protect them from being blamed for missing a diagnosis. This has resulted in what is commonly referred to as defensive medicine. The doctor may just be trying to assure that every possible diagnosis is covered by a test result, even if the diagnosis is highly unlikely. In this way, the doctor cannot be blamed in a malpractice suit for not considering a diagnosis or working up a problem completely. Unfortunately, this practice is necessary to some degree in today's litigious society.

Knowing this, you should ask your doctor what he believes is the likelihood that a given test will help in your diagnosis. If he believes the test will be of marginal help, but admits that he is doing it to cover all possibilities, then you need to decide if you want it done. You can always ask not to have a test done. However, the doctor will most likely want to record your request in your chart, so that it is clear that the test was considered, discussed, and dismissed. This open dialogue between you and your doctor should help to reduce unnecessary tests and their attendant costs, including complications.

STICKER SHOCK!

The best way to control the cost of your work-up is to think about it before the tests are given to you. It is important for you understand why the test is being recommended and don't just take the test out of blind faith or trust. Discuss with your doctor what tests are being ordered and find out how costly they will be. Your doctor may or may not know how much the tests cost. If he doesn't know or gives you a rough estimate, then ask him if there is someone in his billing office or at the lab who would know how much they cost. Once you find out their cost, you might need to schedule another appointment with your doctor to see if the tests are absolutely necessary or ask if there are less expensive alternatives. This approach can be beneficial to you if the treatment is not covered by insurance and you are the one incurring the cost.

Another factor to consider if you want to control costs is comparison shopping. There are some procedures in medicine for which you might want to do some shopping around. For example, it could be to your benefit to shop around for the lowest cost for MRIs, elective surgeries and procedures, and infertility treatments. At the same time, comparison shopping is not appropriate in other instances, for example, if you are suffering a heart attack or have cancer. Also, if your doctor or hospital uses a reference lab for tests, you may not have any choice in who does the test and what it costs. If this is the case, you will just have to accept the cost.

Hopefully if you do your homework, you can find less expensive alternatives or locations for your tests. But remember, cheaper may mean lower quality. Your doctor is usually referring you to a particular doctor or lab because of trust and high quality work. If after questioning your doctor he still strongly suggests you go to the recommended but more expensive doctor or facility, then take your doctor's advice, assuming that you trust him. Your doctor will make a better diagnosis more confidently dealing with other physicians and services that he trusts. The worst thing is to go to the cheaper facility and get the wrong diagnosis that hurts you or delays your care and treatment. Furthermore, a poorly performed test may need to be repeated at the more trusted quality facility. And that may cost you twice as much in the long term.

INSURANCE CONSIDERATIONS

It is important to call your insurance company before you have comprehensive testing to make sure you are covered for the procedure(s). Many plans require preauthorization for some tests, such as MRIs. There are a few exceptions, such as emergency admission, so make sure your insurance will pay for the testing that has been ordered for you.

You should also be aware that day surgery and outpatient procedures at hospitals can be charged by the hour or by the time of day of your scheduled departure (half day, full day, or overnight charges). Therefore, if you stay past your scheduled departure time, it will cost you more. Finally, most insurance companies no longer pay for hospitalization for diagnostic tests unless the person is potentially sick enough to justify being in the hospital in the first place.

WHO ACTUALLY PERFORMS THE TEST?

Some people are surprised when a doctor is not present during the test or diagnostic procedure. The majority of diagnostic tests are actually performed by specialized technicians that are trained in accredited programs to use specific diagnostic and lab equipment and perform the tests. Technicians operate the various ultrasound machines, CAT scanners. and MRI scanners.

It is useful to remember that technicians are not supposed to give out results. Technicians are not trained to make a medical diagnosis, and many a patient has been unnecessarily frightened by a technician attempting to make a diagnosis. All diagnostic tests should be interpreted by a doctor, either your doctor who has ordered the test or a doctor trained specifically to interpret certain types of tests (for example, radiologists, pathologists, cardiologists, or neurologists).

AFTER THE TEST

After a routine test, you will most likely just go home after the test. The doctor's office should provide you with any follow-up test instructions. You may be required to rest for a couple of hours, not drive a vehicle, or take some medication to alleviate any pain or discomfort. Before you leave, ask if there is anything that you are required to do. Knowing this information could save you from post-test complications.

Occasionally, the technician performing the test will recognize something that is abnormal and ask you to wait until he can contact your doctor. The technician needs your doctor to evaluate the test and to decide if you can go home or need further tests. This usually only occurs with some x-ray procedures or possibly with an electro-cardiogram (EKG).

GETTING TEST RESULTS

Look to your main doctor who ordered the test(s) to give you the results. He will also be the one who interprets the results for you. If you call the laboratory or x-ray facility, they will most likely refuse to discuss your tests and instead tell you to contact your doctor. Don't blame the lab for not giving you the results; labs are advised or ordered not to provide you with this information.

The doctor doesn't want you to hear test results from someone who doesn't know your total medical history and who doesn't have a relationship with you. The doctor who orders the test is the one who is responsible for following up on tests and ensuring that appropriate actions are taken. The pathologist, radiologist, and lab technicians just have the responsibility to make sure that your doctor gets the results of the tests. These individuals will not want to directly discuss test results with patients because they usually do not have an ongoing patient/doctor relationship with the patient. Also, in most cases, they do not know the patient nor have complete knowledge of the patients' medical situation.

In the patient/doctor partnership, both individuals assume responsibility for conveying and getting results of tests. It is the doctor's responsibility to inform you of any serious abnormal results. However, it is also your responsibility to find out from him how and when test results will be revealed to you and to make sure you get them. Before the test, you and your doctor should come up with a mutually agreed upon plan for obtaining test results.

As part of your plan, your doctor should indicate an acceptable time frame for when results will be available. Depending on the test, results may be available in minutes or they may take weeks to be determined. However, the norm is that you will have to wait several days for an official report to be generated and sent to the ordering physician. If the doctor needs to base immediate treatment on tests, then he will order them "stat" and the tests will be performed and the results made available as soon as possible.

Different offices have different protocols to handle the vast amounts of test information that they receive daily. Frequently, the technician conducting routine tests will tell you that your doctor will have the results in a certain amount of time. Unfortunately, this time frame isn't always correct. Many patients get upset with the doctor or his staff because the technician mistakenly leads the patient to believe that the result will be available in an hour or the next morning. The technician does not know when the results will be seen and interpreted by your doctor, when the report will get typed, or when the results will be mailed or delivered to you. That is why it is so important to develop a plan with your doctor, so you will know what to expect. If you have not heard from your doctor within the designated time frame, then you should call to find out if the results have arrived yet. If they haven't, get a new time estimate and follow-up again if you need to.

The following are the most common methods for communicating test results:
• via the telephone by either the nurse or doctor,
• via the mail, or
• at a follow-up visit.

If you know ahead of time that you will want a detailed explanation of your results, go ahead and schedule a follow-up visit at the time you schedule the test. If the doctor knows the results could be serious or require complicated choices of treatment, then she will often schedule an appointment to explain the results, present the working diagnosis, and propose a treatment plan. Many test results are best explained with diagrams or pictures or models. This can only be done in the doctor's office during an appointment. It is almost never a waste of time or money to see the doctor to get your test results. After all, it is the best way to get a complete understanding of your diagnosis.

GOOD NEWS—BAD NEWS: WAITING FOR TEST RESULTS

For some, waiting creates almost no anxiety; they expect good news. They believe nothing bad can befall them. It is the nature of others, though, to expect bad news. For them, waiting is an anxious period filled with fear. Still for others, not knowing is the worst part; they want to know even if it's bad news. At least then they can make a plan, take action, and move forward.

Waiting for an important test result can make life seem like it is in limbo—as if you are paused at a crossroads, with two possible futures confronting you. The waiting period is a time filled with powerful emotions and fabricated fears. The emotions attached to waiting are largely governed by whether you see the glass of life as half full or half empty. It is easy to say to yourself, "Don't worry, be happy; focus on the good things in life." But, it is far more difficult to actually follow that advice. If you do have the discipline and willpower to get your mind focused on your work, faith, hobbies, or family, consider it a gift—flow with it. If, however, your emotions win out over your reason in times of stress and you experience that all too human trait called worry, then you may feel that there is no great way to just wait.

There are, however, some good ways to reduce the level of your anxiety and make the waiting period more productive. No single method of waiting works for all individuals. You may need to experiment with the different methods discussed below. In general, go with whatever makes the waiting easier—with two exceptions: We strongly recommend that you avoid elicit drugs and the overuse of alcohol.

Methods to reduce anxiety or add value to the waiting time include:

PRAYER. Can take the form of private prayer at home or public prayer in your house of worship.

MEDITATION. Can yield insight and allay anxiety because it promotes relaxation and clarity of your mind.

EXERCISE. Distracts the mind and gives both a physical and mental energy boost by producing endorphins. Endorphins are morphine-like chemicals that your body produces naturally to give your body and mind a natural lift.

COMMUNICATING. Sharing your fears and anxieties with a friend, loved one, or a professional (psychologist/psychiatrist) is often just enough to help you to better cope with your emotions and situation.

GETTING OUT INTO NATURE. Whether it is taking a walk on the beach or a hike in the woods, nature has a calming influence. It has the quality of returning you to your center.

ENTERTAINMENT. A good way to pass the time and help you to relax is to watch TV or a movie, go to the theater or a sports event, or just listen to your favorite music.

READING. From trashy books to inspirational ones, reading is an effective way to spend quality time with yourself.

POSITIVE THINKING AND VISUALIZATION. Improve your outlook by projecting your image as calm and relaxed with everything ultimately working out.

TOUCH THERAPY. This an important element to relieving anxiety, especially during times of stress. Consider getting a massage, going out dancing, or just plain enjoying what awaits you in the bedroom with a loved one.

SLEEP. Sleep can be curative and restful to the mind and body, as long as it is not a sign of depression.

SHOPPING THERAPY. Whether it's clothes, power tools, or compact disks, it often helps to buy something nice for yourself.

EATING. Food can help, as long as you don't totally overdo it. Small indulgences like hot fudge sundaes may lift your spirits.

WRITING DOWN YOUR THOUGHTS. Keeping a diary or journal can be a powerful tool for reminding yourself what is really important to you.

PREPARING FOR AND GETTING TEST RESULTS

Whatever the outcome of your test results, it may be beneficial for you to focus on the current state of your life. How is your life different from how you wish it to be? Perhaps you will discover insights or changes that will help you better deal with your illness. Then again, maybe your life is exactly where you want it to be. Just being aware of this can serve as a source of inner peace and strength. This in turn might give you the confidence to better deal with your test results. Organize your thoughts, fears, concerns, and expectations as best you can. Take some time to write these thoughts out. Seeing your thoughts on paper is usually more insightful than just thinking them through in your mind.

Test results are returned to doctors in the form of a report. The report will usually include critical values and other relevant statistical information. Your doctor will explain only the relevant values on the report and how they relate to you and your condition. It is also appropriate to ask for a copy of the test results for inclusion in your personal medical files. Additionally, you should write down the doctor's explanation of the results. You may even ask the doctor to write down a brief description of your disease and appropriate reports if you are confused about the diagnosis and test results. This allows you to refer back to them later when you need to refresh your memory. What's more, it helps you to more clearly communicate the results of your tests to your family and friends.

When you get your results, you should also ask for any pamphlets or handouts that your doctor may have about your condition. They can help if you did not fully understand the outcome of the tests or if you missed critical information. If that is the case, then write down your questions. At the next appointment, ask for an explanation. Don't be afraid to pursue this information. It is your body and you have the right know what is going on with it.

ALL TEST HAVE LIMITS

Despite the advances in medical tests, testing remains imperfect. There is no single absolutely perfect test. Errors do occur. The test procedure could be flawed or have limitations, the person performing the test might not do it correctly, or the person interpreting the results might not read them correctly. Additionally, a healthy person who has nothing wrong with him may get an abnormal (positive) test result. This is called a false positive. And a sick person who does have something wrong with him may get a normal (negative) test result. This is called a false negative. As many as 1 out of every 20 test results is estimated to be a false positive or a false negative.

For example, say you go to the doctor and receive a series of tests including a blood sugar. You had a bowl of pasta one hour before the test. Your blood sugar comes back at 180 mg/dl. This is abnormally high and could indicate diabetes. But it also may indicate that you didn't fast as you were told and had too much pasta, which is a starch that turns to sugar in the body. Further testing proves you do not have diabetes. The first test would be a false positive, a test that says you were abnormal when you were not.

It is up to your doctor to determine whether an abnormal result is correct, within the clinical context of your health status. Your doctor must accurately assess your tests and determine whether the abnormal finding fits the symptoms. This is the art of medicine. The mindless acceptance that an abnormal value means certain disease can cause problems for doctors and patients. Doctors must sift out the real abnormalities from the red herrings. Failing to accurately identify the real thing from the impostor leads some doctors off the correct path.

When it comes to interpreting radiological or other imaging techniques, the concept of normal becomes even more complicated. Reading an x-ray or a tissue specimen is not an exercise in numbers or statistics. Here, the patient and ordering physician must rely on the training, experience, and expertise of the reading physician, and question the results if they don't seem to fit. If the reading physician is unsure, he may ask for a second opinion from another reader, or a follow-up study later in time. If uncertainty is involved, it should be stated clearly in the official report.

We cannot stress enough how all tests must be interpreted by your physician in the appropriate clinical context. If the doctor believes you are sick, and all the tests are normal, he must consider the possibility that the tests do not reflect your illness. Alternatively, if he believes you are well, without clinical findings of disease, he must disregard "abnormal" test results that don't make sense. This is the art of medicine.

THE MESSENGER VS. THE MESSAGE!

Being given a test result that you didn't expect or that creates a fearful response can spill over into unjustified anger against the doctor. It may be justifiable to be angry for having a particular problem, but it is not appropriate to be angry at your doctor. After all, your doctor is not the cause of your disease. Instead, he is there to help you identify it, explain it, and treat it.

Work-Up Plan

For each test ordered by your doctor, you should complete the following table. For easier use, enlarge this plan to 200% on a copier.

Name of Test	Date & Time	Location	Who Does the Test	Special Instructions	Advantage/ Disadvantage	Results

1. Before undergoing any test, you should determine if the test is:
   - Technically difficult, painful, and/or poses a risk to your life or well being. If the test poses a real risk, strongly consider the need for the test. Make the doctor justify ordering such an exam.
   - Painful, but safe. If the test is painful but safe, then ask if there is anything that can be done to make the test more comfortable.
   - Expensive. This may prove harmful to your wallet. Ask how the outcome of the test will add to the diagnosis.

2. Ask what will I learn from the test and what will the doctor learn.

3. Write down any additional questions you want to ask the doctor about the test.

Chapter 11

What Is Your Diagnosis?

Charlotte felt tired and run down. At first she thought it was the flu, but after two months her health had not improved. In fact, she was worse. Despite sleeping 12 hours a day, she was still having difficulties concentrating and was falling asleep at work. Some coworkers thought she was depressed; others complained that she had become a lazy slacker. Charlotte had been an outstanding worker and a self-starter during her first three years on the job, so her boss, Martin, knew something must be wrong. He asked Charlotte to go to the doctor.

Tests revealed that she had mononucleosis (mono). Charlotte's mono lasted for 6 months after which she suffered from chronic fatigue syndrome. The prolonged nature of Charlotte's illness required many emotional adjustments. At first, she tried to deny that she was sick. But when it was obvious to her that she was not getting better, she became angry with her illness because it was interfering with her life and career development.

As the chronic fatigue progressed and she grew worse, she worried that she might never recover. She began bargaining with herself. "If only I could get well, I'd stop being so focused on career and take better care of myself." Charlotte became sad and distraught about her situation and how her life had seemed to fall apart.

With time, though, Charlotte's attitude, habits, and life perspective changed. She combined a unique balance of accepting the fact that she was ill while doing all she could to get better. In time, she found herself growing stronger, and soon was back working limited hours. At the same time she was exercising daily and eating well.

After two years, Charlotte finally felt like she had her life back. It was now a more balanced life. Charlotte was very grateful that she had been given a diagnosis because it had helped her understand the changes that were occurring in her body; formulate a treatment plan for recovery; and provide an explanation for her behavior that served as an incentive and justification for her boss to remain understanding and supportive throughout her illness.

Before a diagnosis is known, an illness presents itself as a mystery. After it is known, there is the ability to formulate a treatment regimen and educate those around you about your circumstance. This chapter will help you prepare and deal with your diagnosis.

THE MYSTERY OF THE DIAGNOSIS

It may help you to approach an illness as if you were solving a mystery. A robbery has occurred and your health has been taken. Now you must investigate. Your doctor, in many regards, is your private detective. He culls through your history and examines you and the evidence, looking for clues. The doctor tries to organize and tie together all the clues. The symptoms and physical findings found on examination lead the doctor to what is called a *differential diagnosis*, a list of suspected diseases. Further testing may allow that disease list to become narrowed sufficiently enough to provide a *working diagnosis*. The working diagnosis is the name of the disease most suspected of causing your illness.

What approach does your doctor actually use to come up with his list of diagnoses, since the same constellation of symptoms can be caused by either one or multiple diseases? The intellectual approach used is called the *Principle of Occam's Razor*. Doctors try to explain all of your symptoms as being caused by one disease. For example, you come to your physician with a variety of symptoms, including fatigue, excessive thirst, cold feet, changes in visual acuity, and kidney problems. At first glance it would appear that these multiple symptoms are unrelated and have multiple causes. However, by applying the Principle of Occam's Razor, your physician can explain all of these symptoms as being caused by one underlying disease, diabetes.

The physician first considers each symptom or physical finding individually and then synthesizes the information. This can be confusing to patients because it appears that many different diseases and organ systems are involved. It is the challenge and responsibility of your physician to explain how these multiple symptoms fit together so that you are comfortable that the diagnosis is correct.

At times, all of the symptoms cannot be neatly tied together. If a particular symptom cannot be explained by one disease then your physician needs to consider that either:

- He is not completely familiar with the disease, and the "unexplained" symptom could represent a rare or unusual manifestation of the illness;
- He has the wrong diagnosis; or
- There are multiple diseases causing your symptoms.

With your working diagnosis identified, you and your doctor now begin to test your suspicions. Finding the correct diagnosis may require patience and time as each hypothesized cause is individually examined—sometimes through painstaking trial and error. Diagnostic exams are ordered and treatments prescribed. Your response to treatment is carefully observed. Sometimes, during the course of treatment, new symptoms arise that either confirm or bring into question the working diagnosis. The working diagnosis may change and the process may begin all over until the true culprit, the *final diagnosis*, is determined. And, just as in real life crime stories, some mysteries may never be solved.

THE MOMENT OF DIAGNOSIS

There is power in having your disease identified. Even if you have been sick for days, weeks, or years there is an "uncertain" quality to illness until it is diagnosed. The moment of diagnosis transforms that uncertainty into reality. The words, "You have cancer," or "You have AIDS," have an explosive transforming energy that can change life in an instant. That is why the moment of diagnosis is such a pivotal point in the patient/doctor relationship.

The method by which your doctor tells you about your illness often has far reaching effects, which are frequently under-appreciated by physicians. In fact, many physicians do not even realize that the way they communicate the diagnosis affects the patient's perception of illness. **At the exact moment of diagnosis, what is said, how it is said, and how it is heard creates a strong emotional response that may reverberate throughout the illness.**

A compassionate presentation of the diagnosis may result in hope. A cold, clinical pronouncement of your fate may trigger hopelessness. For example, imagine that you see your family doctor and complain of aches and pains in your joints. He says that you have degenerative arthritis and that it's just one of the many drawbacks of getting older. He further states that there is nothing much that he can do to help you. Feeling depressed by the news and left thinking you are destined to a life of crippling pain, you decide to seek out the advice of a specialist. The rheumatologist paints a different picture. She tells you that there is medicine for the inflammation, she can prescribe a splint for your hand to help you write, and that there are orthopedic shoe pads that help aching feet. She prescribes water aerobics to reduce stress on the body. You leave feeling hopeful that you can improve your outcome. Two doctors treating the same patient and yet providing the patient with two entirely different views of future life with the diagnosis.

Likewise, each patient responds to the diagnosis in a unique and personal manner. Two key factors appear to predetermine a patient's response to illness. The first is the pre-illness attitude toward life and illness. If you have a strong faith in religion, modern medicine, or in your capacity to cure yourself, then you may be better able to weather the knowledge that you have a serious illness. If you have a positive attitude toward life, you may see your diagnosis as a challenge capable of teaching you new lessons. The illness presents an opportunity for personal growth—mentally, emotionally, and spiritually.

On the other hand, if your pre-illness life attitude is negative or you have few emotional or spiritual supports, your diagnosis may create hopelessness or helplessness. You might think there is no way out of your situation.

When your response is negative, you have to confront this pessimism first, before you can confront your illness. This is often a difficult phase because it requires you to develop new attitudes and habits toward life. Once you have a new life view, you can then confront your illness and focus on the treatment and your body's ability to heal itself.

The second factor that contributes to your response is the doctor's method and manner of communicating the diagnosis. Both the words and the way the words are spoken are an important part of the moment of diagnosis. The doctor needs to be cognizant of his effect upon the patient. The patient needs to understand that some doctors hide behind medical terms and Latin words to shield themselves from the pain and awkwardness that is felt at the moment the diagnosis is revealed. Both patient and doctor need to be ever vigilant of the power of words and how communication affects care. The effects of communication are not always immediately identifiable, but they may influence future interactions between patient and doctor. The way in which the doctor and the patient communicate can prove to be the difference between a cure and a bad outcome.

HOW A HEALTH CARE PROVIDER VIEWS A DIAGNOSIS

Depending on the health care provider you visit, your care giver will mostly likely view your diagnosis in different ways. In **western medicine**, doctors are trained to focus on finding the most appropriate diagnosis and then treat the disease or at least slow its progress. The doctor's primary goal is to name the diagnosis and then start treatment. In **alternative medicine**, care givers are trained to focus more on the patient. The goal is to strengthen the patient. This is accomplished by understanding the patient and how the diagnosis impacts the patient's life.

Therefore, the way your provider views the diagnosis will have an impact on how he tells you about the diagnosis and prescribes treatment.

THE NAME GAME

Open a medical textbook and you will find thousands of pages of disease classifications and descriptions. Your **working diagnosis** is the name given to the disease you are thought to have. The name may be very general and incorporate a whole group of symptoms and findings or it may be very specific. For example, chronic fatigue syndrome describes a constellation of signs and symptoms in which overwhelming fatigue is prominent. On the other hand, infectious mononucleosis describes a specific ailment caused by a specific virus (Epstein-Barr), in which fatigue is a central symptom.

Some disease names are categories or subject headings. For example, arthritis is not one disease but hundreds, with many different causes and individual outcomes. Rheumatoid, degenerative, reactive, carcinomatous, and gout are just a few types of arthritis.

Some diseases have generic Latin-based names. For example, hypothyroidism means low thyroid, but the name doesn't tell you how or why it is low. Pharyngitis means inflamed throat, whereas strep pharyngitis tells us that the throat is inflamed with a particular bacterium called streptococcus.

When patients first visit their doctor, they are usually coming to her because they have a complaint or concern and they want to receive preventive care; be relieved from pain; or have a dysfunction fixed. However, ultimately what patients want is to obtain a name for what ails them. Whether it is tracheo-bronchitis, breast cancer, systemic lupus erythematosus, or chronic fatigue syndrome, everyone wants a label that explains and justifies their complaints and symptoms. After all, what do you tell your family when they ask, "What is wrong with you?"

DO YOU UNDERSTAND YOUR DIAGNOSIS?

Because the moment of diagnosis is serious can be emotionally charged, it is not unusual for a patient to hear the diagnosis and then go numb. After hearing your diagnosis and having it translated from DoctorSpeak into English, you should sit back and take some time to reflect on it. Do you understand the diagnosis? Do you believe the diagnosis? What does the diagnosis mean to you and your life?

Even though a diagnosis may be just a single word, it often has many meanings and generates many questions. Gaining mastery over complex problems often involves repetition of information and dividing the information into smaller parts. One way for you to better understand your diagnosis is to look at it in terms of the following four components.

- The scientific name and description of the disease process.
- The practical aspects of the disease as it affects your daily life; physically, mentally, and emotionally.
- The prognosis of the disease (what can you expect in the future?)
- The different treatment options.

By approaching and thinking about your diagnosis in this way, you can begin to understand and incorporate the diagnostic information into a framework that is manageable and meaningful to your life. This approach is easier than trying to understand your entire illness and all of its implications on your life, all at once.

Your doctor, at some point in time, should also discuss with you each of these components of your diagnosis. Thoroughly comprehending all four components of diagnosis will help you to understand and cope with your disease. By completing Exercise 11-1 you can take time to reflect upon what you heard and determine whether you understand it. Sharing this exercise with your doctor may also help to confirm that you do understand your diagnosis.

If after you receive all the information and you are still not comfortable with your diagnosis and cannot accept its accuracy, you may wish to seek a second opinion (Chapter 3). However, before you do extensive retesting or see numerous doctors, you may need to consider the possibility that you are in denial. This is especially true if your diagnosis is onerous.

HOW DOES YOUR DIAGNOSIS AFFECT YOUR LIFE?

The sounds of certain words like cancer, AIDS, and Alzheimer's bring fear into the hearts of even the strongest individuals. Don't expect that you will be able to hear the news of your illness and immediately be in full acceptance of it. It may take some time getting used to the idea of having a "disease." Dr. Elisabeth Kübler-Ross in the book *On Death and Dying* describes the emotional stages that a dying patient passes through. These stages are also applicable to the disease process because disease in many ways represents the death of wellness.

DENIAL OR DISBELIEF: *"This can't be happening to me!"* Denial and disbelief help protect you mentally and emotionally from the pain of reality. It is perfectly normal to deny your illness; every patient experiences denial at one time or another. You can pretend there is no problem and that your life will soon return to normal. Unfortunately, or fortunately, you can't keep the denial up forever. At some point, you need to recognize your denial so that you don't prolong your illness or delay recovery.

ANGER: *"This isn't fair!"* You may find yourself directing your anger toward your friends, family, and the medical establishment. However, your anger is usually not directly related to anything they have done. Instead, your anger is more about having your life interrupted by this disease and perhaps not being able to complete your goals or enjoy your life as much as you would like.

BARGAINING: *"I promise to... , if I am only cured."* Bargaining is trying to make deals with yourself, your God, or your doctor in hopes of curing your illness or extending your life. Most bargains are quite personal and usually kept to yourself or God or your clergy.

DEPRESSION: *"I'll never be happy and/or well again."* The old saying is that it is usually darkest before the dawn. You might have difficulty functioning on a daily basis during this phase. But it is also during this stage that you must acknowledge your illness. When you can no longer deny your illness, you can begin to mourn your losses. You can expect to react to the loss of your health, both past and future, and to the impending loss of your old way of life. It is OK to be depressed because it allows you to fully experience your sorrow and grief and to move onto acceptance.

ACCEPTANCE: *"I know I have the strength to face my illness. My doctor and I will do our best and I intend to enjoy the good days as much as possible."* **VS. RESIGNATION:** *"What's the use, my life is miserable and I suffer. There is nothing my doctor or I can do about it."* This is the final stage of illness. There is an important difference between acceptance and resignation.

Acceptance is facing reality and its many possible outcomes with an inner peace and strength. It involves moving toward health. By using your energies for repair rather than internal conflict, your mind and body can enhance your healing capacity. **Acceptance is not the absence of fear; however, it is finding the courage to master fear.** Acceptance does not guarantee wellness, but it does offer you the best chance you have for healing.

Resignation differs significantly from acceptance. Resignation is giving up. A patient who is resigned to being ill and not getting better may feel overwhelmed by the disease and treatment. For example, there seems to be so many steps to getting better that you don't know where to begin. Patients can become resigned to being ill because of being paralyzed by fear. You may be afraid of losing control of your body or mind. You might be afraid of being less than you were before your illness and not being able to care for yourself or your family. You might be frightened by the unknown pain and suffering associated with disease or you may be afraid of dying.

Whatever your fear, explore it, even though it may be painful. This will help you with accepting your illness. You may discover a peace of mind that will assist you in progressing through all of the emotional stages of illness. Being at peace with your body and mind may also have a healing capacity. Today, many physicians, scientists, and philosophers believe the mind-body connection has potent curative powers. Exercise 11-2 will help you to determine your current state of mind.

THE ILLNESS PARADIGM

You may hope that your illness will not dramatically change your life. But the reality is, illness changes lives. Not only does illness change your physical life but it may also change your perspective on life, your paradigm. Your paradigm is your view of the world. It is influenced by your life's past and present experiences. A paradigm is analogous to looking at the world through a pair of glasses. If you are healthy, your glasses may be clear or rose colored. You live in a paradigm of health and for you the world is physically comfortable and rosy.

But when you become ill your paradigm shifts. A new paradigm, an illness paradigm, is created. The lens through which you perceive the world becomes distorted. Activities that were once easy and painless become more difficult and painful (physically or mentally). You may be challenged by new obstacles, fears, or doubts.

To better understand your present focus, there is a question you may wish to ask yourself.

ARE YOU (1) A PERSON FOCUSING ON LIFE WHO HAPPENS TO HAVE AN ILLNESS, OR (2) A PERSON FOCUSING ON ILLNESS WHO HAPPENS TO HAVE A LIFE?

If your illness is severe enough, you may have to readjust your focus. There are many paths around obstacles. After all, there are blind skiers and partially paralyzed rock climbers. You can have a positive impact on your state of mind and disease just by choosing to focus on what is still great in your life.

INSIDER'S HINT
....

"You see things and you say, 'Why?' but I dream things that never were and say, 'Why not?'"—George Bernard Shaw

The illness paradigm does not only affect you but it also greatly affects others in your life. It may take time for family members and friends to adjust; they may not be capable of understanding your point of view if they have never had a serious illness. After all, they are still viewing life through the paradigm of health. You and they have been thrust into a new situation. To help your relationships survive an illness, you will all be required to use genuine communication, have a positive attitude, practice forgiveness, and focus on hope and understanding.

One thing is certain, a serious illness challenges all and forces all to adapt. Patients, friends, and families who embrace life, despite illness, have the power to heal and serve as inspirations to others. Exercise 11-3 will help you to bring into focus your current illness paradigm.

THE FAILURE TO ACCURATELY DIAGNOSE YOUR ILLNESS

The inability to accurately diagnose an illness is a common reason that patients do not improve or that treatment fails. As we have mentioned, medicine is an art not a precise science. The very phrase the "practice of medicine" reflects the less than exact nature of that art. The act of cataloguing information in medical journals, the requirements for continuing medical education, and years of intense schooling are all attempts to share the combined knowledge of medicine's practitioners.

Despite all these attempts to make practitioners perfect and medicine more precise, mistakes and limitations in knowledge exist—in part, because the information in the field of medicine is ever expanding and the response to disease from individual to individual rarely identical. As a result, one of the most difficult aspects of medicine is making the correct diagnosis, and then based on the diagnosis, devising the correct treatment plan.

It is important to recognize this imperfection in medicine and be prepared to deal with the reality that you may be given no diagnosis or an incorrect diagnosis. The following are some common diagnostic dilemmas.

YOUR DOCTOR KNOWS HE IS UNABLE TO MAKE THE DIAGNOSIS. This is when a series of symptoms do not make sense to your doctor. An example of this is a 43-year-old woman who has swollen lymph nodes, a fever, and fatigue. All routine tests indicate that an illness is present. The preliminary diagnosis is a cancerous lymphoma. A biopsy of the enlarged nodes is performed and is inconclusive. However, the primary care doctor is uncomfortable with that diagnosis because of the inconclusive nature of the tests. The woman is sent to a university where it is discovered that she has Cat Scratch Fever, an infection that mimics lymphoma. The Cat Scratch Fever is treated with antibiotics and the patient is cured. The initial diagnosis of cancer created a great sense of concern and worry for the woman and her family. The wrong treatment could have been implemented had her primary care doctor not sent her for a second opinion.

INSIDER'S HINT
....

Give credit to your doctor when she knows her limits and sends you for extra testing or for a second opinion. If your doctor can't make a diagnosis in a reasonable time period, ask to see a specialist for a second opinion.

YOUR DOCTOR MAKES THE WRONG DIAGNOSIS. Not surprisingly, a constellation of symptoms may lead your doctor to the wrong diagnosis. An example of this is a 70-year-old woman who has excruciating stomach pains for one month. She is a stoic woman and reliable historian. Her doctor tells her that she probably has an ulcer induced by stress, but no tests are performed to confirm the diagnosis. He prescribes Maalox. For two months the pain continues to get worse. She calls her doctor again and again, and he orders a stronger prescription but still no diagnostic tests. Finally, the pain sends the woman to the emergency room where another doctor orders an ultrasound of the abdomen which reveals a cancer of the pancreas, metastatic to liver.

This patient's final outcome likely was not altered by the delay in diagnosis because pancreatic cancer is often not cured unless caught extremely early. Still, for other cancers, a missed diagnosis can result in delay of treatment which is troubling because of the physical and the emotional pain it creates in the lives of the patients. At its worst, a missed diagnosis can result in a prolongation of treatment, disability, or loss of life that might not have occurred if an accurate diagnosis had been made.

A doctor may tell a patient that a problem is emotional and all in his head. It's true that many problems are psychological in nature or stress induced. But if the problem turns out to be physical and the patient was told it was emotional, the doctor-patient relationship is usually irreparably damaged.

INSIDER'S HINT
....

It is imperative that you insist that appropriate diagnostic tests be performed before a conclusion is reached that the problem is psychological.

A NAME IS GIVEN TO THE ILLNESS BUT THE CAUSE IS POORLY UNDERSTOOD (POORLY UNDERSTOOD ILLNESSES). The cause and effect of most illnesses is relatively well understood. The diagnosis of most afflictions can be accurately named and a treatment prescribed. However, during the earliest years of a new outbreak or when a condition has many causes, it is not uncommon for the diagnosis to be given a "catch-name" yet not be well understood.

In the 1970s women began to go into shock for unknown reasons. As the cases accumulated it was realized that the onset of symptoms was during menses (periods). At first, doctor's were puzzled as to the cause; but within months they learned that all these women had a common vaginal infection. Later they discovered the cause and source of the infection was a new type of tampon that was being used incorrectly. They called the condition toxic shock. The name was given to the disease even before it was fully understood. This sequence of events is representative of many new epidemics.

Throughout history the introduction of new chemicals, machines, and infectious agents into the environment have resulted in new diseases, most of which are at first poorly understood. The first individuals afflicted are often disbelieved and mistreated. These early sufferers are frequently diagnosed as malingerers, hysterical, or crazy. Only after time, and after the disease has affected many more people, is the cause of the illness revealed. This has been true in the past for lead poisoning, mercury poisoning, silicosis, radiation induced cancer, asbestosis, cigarette smoking, DDT/pesticide induced diseases, repetitive stress injuries, recurrent ulcers (H Pylori) and AIDS to name just a few conditions.

Today we have no good explanation for the Gulf War illness, multiple chemical sensitivity, or chronic fatigue. Medicine, big business, and the government have denounced and delegitimized these conditions and degraded the sufferers by initially labeling them all as kooks, fakes, phonies, and psychosomatics.

History suggests that a cause and an explanation will be found for these Poorly Understood Illnesses.

INSIDER'S HINT

If you suffer from a Poorly Understood Illness, it is important to persevere, remain proactive, and realize that the resistance and demeaning attitude you encounter usually arises from the limitations of science and the political or monetary concerns of government and business. Find a doctor who is sympathetic, and work with her to find a treatment that works for you.

BEWARE OF DR. KNOW-IT-ALL

Know-it-all doctors are most frequently doctors who feel like it is them against the world. Normally doctors work together and help each other solve difficult problems. But some doctors are unwilling or unable to consistently work together with their colleagues. Their inability to cooperate with their medical associates may prove dangerous to your health. You may wish to avoid these doctors. An example of such a doctor is the neurosurgeon who rejects and will not communicate to you another doctor's opinion, if it differs from his. His pat answer may be "they don't know what they're doing" because he believes that he alone knows the correct solution to your problem.

There is a fine line between confidence and arrogance. Confidence should include a willingness to listen, answer difficult questions, and logically communicate a personal opinion even if it should prove contradictory to the majority viewpoint.

Warning signs that should alert you that a doctor is carrying excess baggage include:

• Doctors who put down their colleagues
• Doctors who consistently tell you not to trust anyone else's opinion
• Doctors who refuse or are strongly against you seeking a second opinion
• Doctors who refuse to explain outside or contradictory opinions
• Doctors who consistently refuse to listen to you, their staff, or their colleagues
• Doctors who behave as if they know it all

HOW CAN YOU EDUCATE YOURSELF FURTHER?

It is your body, your life, and your disease. You will ultimately be responsible for ensuring that you receive the proper diagnosis and care. You can best do this with knowledge. The worst thing you can do is crawl into a hole. There are almost limitless educational resources available. Knowledge and information are available from your doctor, local libraries, and now the Internet (see Chapter 4).

Perhaps the most-user friendly source of information can be obtained from **support groups** specific to your disease (for example, a local breast cancer support group). These volunteer, non-profit groups meet regularly and offer both verbal and written materials that are patient oriented. They provide technical, informational, and emotional support from others who have dealt with or are dealing with the same issues as you. These support groups reinforce the notion that you are not alone in your struggle. Within these groups you will meet some individuals whose illnesses are worse and others whose illnesses are cured or in remission.

Being exposed to these individuals can create a swirl of emotions, including fear, gratitude, jealousy, anxiety, and hope. These emotions, even those that feel negative, are very human and are best felt and expressed. You may even secretly wish others to get ill, even for one day, just to better understand your plight. If you confront these emotions in yourself with the aid of a support group, you can utilize these feelings to empower yourself. By using the past and present experiences of others to educate yourself, and adopting and emulating (modeling) some of the techniques that work for others, you will catalyze the process of self acceptance and optimize your chances for wellness. You may even uncover a means to diagnosis and treat your illness.

WHAT'S NEXT?

It is not just the diagnosis that determines the outcome or prognosis of your illness. Instead, it is a combination of the disease you have, the effectiveness of your treatment, and the response of your mind and body to that treatment. In Chapter 13, the concept of prognosis will be discussed. Before that, in Chapter 12, we will review a variety of treatment issues and options.

EXERCISE 11-1

Understanding Your Diagnosis

1. What is your diagnosis? _____

_____

_____

_____

_____

2. What does the diagnosis mean to you? _____

_____

_____

3. Do you believe the diagnosis? Why do you believe or not believe the diagnosis? _____

_____

_____

4. How does your diagnosis affect your daily life? _____

_____

_____

5. What is your prognosis? The likely outcome of your diagnosis? ___

_____

_____

6. What are your options for getting better (treatment options)? ___

_____

_____

7. Is there anything you do not understand about your diagnosis? ___

_____

_____

8. If you answer yes to question 7: What questions should you ask your doctor in order to better understand your diagnosis? _____

_____

_____

EXERCISE 11-2

Your Emotional Stage

Which stage best describes your current emotional state of mind? For each attribute under each stage, rate your emotion on a scale of 0 to 5 (with 0 = do not feel this way, 3 = feel this way sometimes, and 5 = feel this way all of the time. Total the individual attribute scores to determine an emotional stage score. The stage with the highest score is your primary state of mind at this point in time.

DENIAL/DISBELIEF

___ Cannot believe this is happening to you.

___ Believe test results may be inaccurate.

___ Believe that you don't need to take the treatment or medications.

___ You find yourself pretending that you are not ill while around other people.

___ **Total Denial Score**

ANGER

___ Feel that life isn't fair.

___ Find yourself getting upset with your doctor, family, or friends.

___ Feel envious of well people.

___ Feel bitter about things you should or shouldn't have done to prevent this illness.

___ **Total Anger Score**

BARGAINING

___ Find yourself making deals with God.

___ Find yourself making deals with yourself.

___ Find yourself making deals with the doctor and other medical staff.

___ Set goals for recovery.

___ **Total Bargaining Score**

EXERCISE 11-2

Your Emotional Stage *(cont.)*

DEPRESSION

___ Find that you cannot get through your daily routine.

___ Find that your eating and sleeping habits have changed.

___ Don't feel like socializing with family or friends.

___ Feel sad, gloomy, helpless, or hopeless.

___ **Total Depression Score**

ACCEPTANCE

___ Have acknowledged the reality of your diagnosis.

___ Feel prepared to handle your treatment.

___ Feel that you can handle changes in your daily life.

___ Feel that you have the strength to cope with your illness.

___ **Total Acceptance Score**

RESIGNATION

___ Feel fearful about your health.

___ Feel fearful about your future.

___ Recognize your fate, but are not able to accept it.

___ Believe treatment is a process you must get through, and
expect little hope for the future.

___ **Total Resignation Score**

Describe why you think you are at your current emotional stage.

_____

_____

_____

_____

_____

Describe how you can get through this stage.

_____

_____

_____

_____

_____

EXERCISE 11-3

What Is Your Illness Paradigm?

Not only does illness change your physical life, but it may also change your perspective on life—your paradigm. By analyzing the circumstances of your illness, and how you've reacted to it all, you can start the emotional aspect of healing.

1. HOW? WHY? WHEN? WHERE? WHAT?

a. How sick are you? _____

_____

b. Why did you get sick? _____

_____

c. When did you get sick? _____

_____

d. Where did you get sick? _____

_____

e. What are the predisposing factors that lead to you getting sick? _

_____

2. Check one: Do you view yourself as:

____a person focused on life who happens to have an illness? or

____a person focused on illness who happens to have a life?

3. Why do you view yourself in this manner?_____

_____

_____

_____

_____

4. Specifically, how would you describe your attitude toward your:

Life: _____

Health: _____

Faith: _____

Fear: _____

EXERCISE 11-3

What Is Your Illness Paradigm? *(cont.)*

5. How have your friends and family responded and adapted to your diagnosis?
You may wish to ask them to read and comment on your answer.

_____

_____

_____

_____

_____

_____

_____

_____

6. What can you do now and in the next few days to feel more educated and empowered about your diagnosis?

_____

_____

_____

_____

_____

_____

_____

Chapter 12

Treatment and Healing

Mildred had been healthy all of her 57 years. She had never smoked, only drank socially, and was never overweight. So it was a shock when her family practice physician, Dr. Thomas, told her that she had colon cancer. He immediately referred her to an oncologist (a cancer specialist) who suggested that with chemotherapy, radiation, and possibly limited surgery she had an excellent chance for a full recovery.

Mildred was afraid of cancer. But she was even more fearful of the side effects associated with cancer treatment. When she returned to Dr. Thomas, she asked him to outline her treatment options, including some less drastic alternative therapies. He outlined three basic choices:
- Do nothing and let nature take its course, or
- Undergo traditional chemotherapy and radiation treatment, or
- Go on a macrobiotic diet to "strengthen the immune system" to naturally fight the cancer.

Mildred chose the macrobiotic diet. Three months later, she felt worse and visited the oncologist rather than Dr. Thomas. After further testing, he informed Mildred that her cancer had grown dramatically. He asked what form of therapy she and Dr. Thomas had chosen. She reported that she had religiously followed the prescription for the alternative macrobiotic diet. She couldn't understand why it hadn't worked better. To Mildred, alternative meant different but equally effective. She had wanted to believe the macrobiotic diet would work, and because it had been presented by an M.D. she never questioned whether it had ever been proven effective.

The oncologist remained silent but was upset for Mildred because she had probably lost her best chance for a cure. During the three month interval the cancer had invaded her bladder. Liver metastases had also developed. If chemotherapy, radiation, and/or surgical treatment were attempted now, it would have to be very aggressive including extensive surgery in which her bladder and rectum would be removed. This would likely leave Mildred incapacitated.

The oncologist was distressed that Dr. Thomas had presented and prescribed an unproved alternative method of treatment as if it were a proven method. Dr. Thomas had not properly informed the patient of the different outcomes for the various treatments. There is no evidence that a macrobiotic diet is any better for colon cancer than receiving no care at all. Perhaps the deception was unintentional but it was concerning that Dr. Thomas who is a strong believer and crusader for alternative medicine, had allowed his bias to negatively affect Mildred's life.

Mildred has not only lost much of her faith in alternative medicine, but she may also lose her life. She now is returning to traditional (allopathic) medicine for help, but it may be too little too late.

Tonya had a different experience with traditional and alternative medicine. A licensed nurse practitioner who practices traditional Western medicine, Tonya was 35 years old when she began experiencing headaches. Because they grew more intense, she visited her doctor, who ordered an MRI scan. The radiologist found a small cystic fluid collection along the top of her brain. The cyst created no pressure or harm to the brain. Still, her doctor was concerned that this could be causing the headaches. Urgent surgery was performed and the fluid drained. This did not solve the headache problem. Shortly after the surgery, the fluid re-accumulated. Tonya sought a second opinion regarding the fluid collection. She was advised that it should be left alone and that it was not the cause of the headaches.

The headaches persisted until she was treated for a sinus infection. Over the next three years, Tonya had several unpleasant and unsatisfying experiences with traditional medicine, mostly side effects from medications and back pain. She often felt her doctors were in too much of a hurry to take the time to hear her needs. In response to her frustration, she began exploring naturopathy, massage, and acupuncture therapy. Her sinuses and back pain improved dramatically.

Although Tonya still practices nursing and recognizes the value of traditional Western medicine, she is an advocate of combining alternative and western medicine.

TREATMENT APPROACHES AND PHILOSOPHIES

As you have read, there is wisdom and limitations of traditional western and alternative medicine. And when planning your treatment, it is useful to develop a philosophy that will guide you through your illness. This philosophy should incorporate both resolve and resilience. Treatment cannot be constantly changing with each setback, nor should it be inflexible in the face of persistent failure. The following provides a framework for integrating the best of allopathic and alternative medicine into your daily care.

TRADITIONAL WESTERN MEDICINE (ALLOPATHY) focuses on the disease. It approaches illness from the perspective that there is a disease invading the body which is causing an otherwise healthy person to become ill. Traditional western medicine strives to identify the disease and either treat its symptoms (for example, insulin for diabetes and narcotics for back pain) or when possible, eradicate the disease (for example, surgery for a herniated disc).

When the focus is eradicating disease, the treatments can be invasive and out of harmony with body. When attacking a disease, western medications and surgery sometimes end up attacking the patient's body as much as it attacks the disease. We experience this as side effects. For example, antibiotics kill bacteria in the throat but also create diarrhea by killing the healthy bacterial flora in the colon. Chemotherapy kills cancer cells but it also kills healthy cells such as hair follicles, mucous membranes, and important natural immune cells.

Destructive diseases such as cancer require powerful intervention in order to be cured. For these illnesses, traditional Western medicine is usually the treatment of choice despite its undesirable side effects. For Mildred, surgery and chemotherapy may have saved her life. Although alternative medicine including improved diet and stress reduction may have assisted in recovery, they were not appropriate first lines of therapy and were not a substitute for chemotherapy, surgery, and radiation.

ALTERNATIVE MEDICINE focuses on restoring balance to the body. It approaches illness from the perspective that there is an imbalance or loss of harmony, a *dis-ease,* within the body which is causing the person to become ill. Alternative medicine focuses on reducing stress and strengthening the body's natural healing forces. It strives to identify and treat that imbalance (for example, acupuncture for back pain and chiropractic manipulation for muscular-skeletal mechanical back pain).

Alternative medicine provides methods for daily living that are in harmony with the body. Since it is estimated that up to 90 percent of illnesses of modern society are stress and lifestyle related, alternative medicine which focuses on these elements of living is gaining popularity. Its many teachings emphasize balance through proper diet, rest, and exercise. Disciplines such as yoga, meditation, and massage are as much a way to live as they are therapies. Alternative medicine accentuates reducing stress, maintaining body-mind strength through balance, and returning homeostasis to the whole, when body functions arc perturbed. It is believed that healing is facilitated (the immune system, for example, is improved) when a balanced and healthy mind-body connection is maintained. This helps to fight and prevent disease. If disease should strike, the body is better prepared to recover.

For many people, alternative medicine is attractive simply because it is not traditional medicine. There is the perception that alternative medicine is natural, harmonious, and safer to the body while western medicine is synthetic, discordant, and dangerous to the body. Also there is the sense for some people that they control their care and medical destiny to a greater degree in alternative medicine than in western medicine. In Tonya's case, she found relief with alternative solutions after traditional medicine had failed her.

THE NEW MEDICINE: INTEGRATED MEDICINE
Medicine is evolving and giving birth to a new form of medicine, integrated medicine. We use the term integrated medicine to mean combining Western principles of diagnosis (identifying disease) and treatment (eradicating disease and treating symptoms) with alternative medicine's approach of strengthening and treating the whole person. Integrated medicine blurs the boundaries between traditional Western medicine and alternative care. Today, diet and exercise are as much a part of controlling heart disease as are cholesterol lowering medications and CABG surgery (coronary artery bypass grafts).

New less-invasive procedures for treating cancer such as prostate seed implantation radiation treatment are replacing radical prostatectomy surgery. New limited surgeries (laparoscopy) and catheter procedures (angioplasty) are being employed in place of old surgical procedures. These minimally invasive procedures are less of an insult to the body and thus allow the individual to recuperate more quickly. The following story illustrates how integrated medicine can work.

After a climbing accident Tim had a huge herniated disc for which he received surgery. He did great for five years until he reinjured his back and started to again suffer from muscle spasms, and back and leg pain. He had developed degenerative changes in the region of the surgery and had a mild reherniation of the remnant disc material. His doctors advised against surgery. Instead, they recommended an integrated medical approach of routine anti-inflammatory medication, physical therapy, massage, acupuncture, meditation, a graduated exercise and weight program, and traditional medications for acute flair-ups (steroids and muscle relaxers, for example). Although not pain free, Tim has gone from limited activity with constant pain to a near normal activity level with controllable symptoms.

INSIDER'S HINT:

It is not necessary to use a cannon to kill a flea. It is also unwise to attempt to stop a charging tiger with a fly swatter. (Yes, you could get lucky, but do you really want to take that chance with your life?)

When invasive procedures and medications are required for a cure they should be utilized. But it is not necessary to use a cannon to kill a flea. If a disease is less serious, consider using less invasive therapy if it is reasonably well documented to be effective and do no harm. The challenge facing doctors and patients today is knowing how and when and which combination of medical therapies to apply.

The correct therapeutic regimen for each patient is highly dependent upon the disease, the person and their beliefs, as well as the circumstances of the illness. Sometimes traditional therapy is more appropriate, while at other times, alternative therapy may prove to be the treatment of choice. Alternative and allopathic medicine need not be viewed as mutually exclusive. Instead, in most cases they can be applied together, in parallel to function synergistically (additively). That approach means utilizing and integrating the best that traditional and alternative care have to offer.

RETURNING TO OUR HIPPOCRATIC ROOTS

In many ways, when Western medicine applies the principles of integrated medicine it is returning to its traditional roots. The philosophy of treating the whole person is not a departure from traditional Western medicine but rather a return to its basic Hippocratic roots.

Hippocrates, the father of modern western medicine, lived at about the time of 400 BC, when many patients died of illnesses that today are routinely cured. Still, some patients treated by Hippocrates were able to naturally combat illness through diet, rest, and herbal remedies. Many of the ancient lessons of healing have been forgotten which if applied today might prove beneficial.

Hippocrates is among the most respected ancient healers. He advocated four fundamental principles known as the Hippocratic code. They apply as much today as they did 2000 years ago. But because doctors in the 21st century have such vastly superior tools and knowledge with which to cure patients, they sometimes forget to apply Hippocrates' most basic principles.

1. Observe carefully. This allows the doctor to properly identify the patient's disease and response to treatment.
2. Know the patient. This allows the doctor to prescribe a treatment that is in harmony with the patient and the patient's lifestyle.
3. Evaluate honestly and use diet and nature's remedies to strengthen the body. In ancient times there were few medicines. It was vital to use natural healing powers to strengthen the body through rest, diet, and exercise.
4. Treat cautiously—do no harm. This acknowledges the awareness that the doctor has powerful remedies which can harm or kill the patient. Hippocrates warned doctors to weigh the benefit of medical intervention against its risk.

Modern advances in surgery, medicine, and diagnostic testing eclipse the skills of Hippocrates. These breakthroughs have been accomplished because during the last 200 years researchers have systematically and scientifically focused on what causes disease. Advances in surgical techniques, immunizations, antibiotics, treatment medications, imaging scanners, and chemotherapy and radiation therapy assist people in living longer and healthier lives.

By the mid 20th century, it appeared that if modern medicine continued to expand at its incredible rate it might cure cancer and eliminate most diseases. Perhaps, patients began expecting "magic bullet" cures and doctors, impressed by their knowledge and powerful achievements, anticipated finding newer and more potent cures.

Despite incredible achievements, there are still diseases that we cannot cure (viruses such as HIV/AIDS); treatments that work for some but not for others (failed back surgery); and old diseases once controlled that have mutated and discovered new ways to defeat the "modern miracle cures" (tuberculosis developing antibiotic resistance).

The byproduct of these modern breakthroughs has been that the focus of Western medicine has swung toward treating diseases and away from treating patients. Fortunately, there is a new awareness that there are limitations to just treating diseases without focusing attention on treating the individual patient's needs. We recommend the combined approach, integrated medicine, be part of your treatment plan.

CHOOSING A TREATMENT PROGRAM

After your diagnosis your doctor should outline a treatment plan. This is a logical course of action prescribed to treat your condition. Whether it is simple or complex, you should not leave your doctor's office without understanding the plan. If necessary, ask to have the plan written out for you. Also ask your doctor any questions you have concerning the plan. If you need some time to think about the plan and its implications, do not hesitate to let your doctor know.

The treatment plan must take into account whether the disease is acute or chronic; benign or malignant; curable or incurable; life threatening or life altering. It should reflect whether you wish to treat the illness yourself or obtain assistance. It should address whether that assistance will include traditional and/or alternative providers.

Approaching your treatment plan in an organized manner should help to keep you from becoming overwhelmed with the many options that are available.

KEYS TO CHOOSING AN EFFECTIVE TREATMENT PLAN

1. Understand each component of the plan and why it is being utilized.

2. Consider all treatment options with an open mind.

3. Educate yourself regarding each treatment option.

4. Ask your caregiver about the pros and cons of each treatment.

5. Decide which treatments are correct for you.

6. Monitor closely the effectiveness of each treatment.

7. Adjust and add treatments as warranted.

8. Approach treatment with a positive proactive self-caring attitude.

9. Examine and work to heal the aspects of your physical, spiritual, and emotional life that are out of balance.

MEASURING THE EFFECTIVENESS OF YOUR TREATMENT STRATEGIES

As you well know, the usual reason why people go to a doctor when they have a problem is simple—to get well. The effectiveness of a healer is determined by the effectiveness of the treatment. For most people, a doctor is good if she can effectively treat the illness and relieve any suffering. She is great if she can cure the illness and prevent recurrence.

Of course, some but not all conditions can be cured. For some illnesses, the symptoms can be controlled, as is the case with diabetes. For other conditions, symptoms may be well controlled most of the time but intermittently flair-up and cause great discomfort and interference with lifestyle (back pain after lifting or strenuous gardening).

TREATMENT EFFECTIVENESS YARDSTICKS
  • Control of pain
  • Restoration of an impaired body function
  • Prevention

PAIN is the body's warning signal that something is wrong. But when pain becomes severe enough, it can interfere with normal function. Pain can take the joy out of life and become debilitating. Treatment can be directed at covering up the pain (with narcotics, for example), reducing the cause of the pain and strengthening the body (with massage, physical therapy, or acupuncture), and/or eliminating the underlying problem (herniated disc or hip replacement surgery).

IMPAIRED BODY FUNCTION occurs when any part of the body is not operating at normal efficiency. Often it shuts down to protect itself from further harm. But when dysfunction becomes too severe it can become life threatening. Treatments directed at restoring body function can take the form of compensating for the disease (insulin for diabetes), strengthening the body and mind (meditation and yoga to relieve stress) and curing the underlying problem (antibiotics to treat bacterial pneumonia). Exercise 12-1 can help you assess your treatment plan's level of success.

PREVENTION can be directed at preventing an illness from developing or treating a condition early before it becomes harmful. When attempting to prevent an illness from developing you may either:

- Know that you are at risk for a specific condition. For example, if your mother and aunt had breast cancer, you will need to be more vigilant than others regarding self examinations, physician examinations, and screening mammograms. You should start these screening programs much earlier than an individual who is not at risk. There are many known conditions that are associated with illnesses (for example, inherited birth defects and genetic predisposition for certain diseases, smoking-related cancer, and HIV from unprotected intercourse).
- Not know that you are at risk for a specific condition. Some illnesses develop for which you have no family history or predisposing factors. For example, even if no one in their family has had prostate cancer, it is wise for men to go in for a routine screening exam every year after age 50. This screening exam should include a digital exam and PSA (prostate specific antigen) test. If an abnormality is detected, a prostate biopsy is warranted. It is the objective of early detection and treatment to identify and eliminate disease early when it is curable, before any irreversible damage has occurred.

INSIDER'S HINT
....
Prevention and early treatment are the best forms of treatment.

OUTCOMES OF TREATMENT

Illnesses may develop and disappear quickly or they may linger chronically. Dealing with your illness may simulate a sprint or marathon. You will need to prepare yourself for the challenge. The usefulness of any given treatment is a combination of its medical effectiveness, the confidence you have that it will work, and your willingness to follow through with treatment (compliance).

COMPLETE CURE is a cherished outcome of all treatments. There is often a difference between recovery and cure. Alcoholics are recovered but they are not cured. They require constant discipline to prevent their disease from recurring. The same principle applies to individuals with conditions like stroke or a prior heart attack.

CURE implies that the disease is eradicated, but it does not mean it cannot recur. If your child has an ear infection and receives antibiotics he may be fully cured. However, the shape of the ear canal may predispose him to recurrent new infections.

Cure and recovery are thus conditional. In order to know that an illness is truly cured, it requires time. If you do not have a recurrence of an illness such as cancer within five to seven years you are considered cured. To ensure the best long-term outcome (prognosis), we recommend vigilance and preventive care even in the midst of apparent recovery and cure.

REMISSION is when the disease is no longer detectable or symptomatic within the body. Treatment appears to have been effective. For some people, the remission is the first sign of a complete recovery and cure. But for others, the disease lies hidden within the body waiting to re-emerge. Herpes or cancer can lie dormant for weeks or years undetectable until some form of stress or damage to the body's defenses triggers the illness' recurrence.

RECURRENCES AND RELAPSES represent the return of a disease and its symptoms. A recurrence or relapse is one of the most frustrating aspects of illness. It steals hope. Just as you are feeling better and getting confidence that you are well—boom—you're sick again. It takes courage and perseverance to begin the treatment process all over again.

The words *recurrence* and *relapse* are commonly applied to cancer and infections. For both infections and cancers, the same treatment is often less effective the second time around. This is because the original cancer cells or the bacteria have mutated (changed) and become resistant to treatment. For these recurrent conditions, newer, more expensive, and often more toxic drugs or measures are required to control the disease.

For most other conditions, a recurrence can be treated by applying the same treatment principles that initially worked (with gout, for example, taking the medications, avoiding high-purine foods, and refraining from alcohol). Still, for some diseases or conditions, especially those that were initially treated with surgery, a second surgery or similar treatment is less effective. For example, attempts to treat a reherniated disc with surgery a second time have a less favorable prognosis, so lifestyle changes may be the only solution.

INSIDER'S HINT
....

Recurrence and relapse can steal your hope. It takes courage and perseverance to begin the treatment process all over again,

PREVENTION should be a part of all treatment plans. This involves planning how not to get sick as well as preventing recurrences. Prevention applies to simple things like strains and sprains as well as complex illnesses such as cancer, stroke, and heart attacks, which require lifestyle changes such as stopping smoking. Treatment plans should include preventive care that is specific for your condition.

Even if you are not yet cured it is useful to incorporate the habits required for prevention. We recognize that you may not be able to completely prevent a recurrence of your cancer, but if you are alert you can detect it early and more likely treat it effectively. Appendix 2 lists recommendations for maximizing prevention and optimizing wellness.

DO YOU AGREE WITH THE TREATMENT PLAN?

In addition to understanding the plan, you also need to agree with the treatment prescribed. If you do not see the logic in the plan, be persistent and ask your doctor for more information on the options available to you. Ask why he has specifically recommended the particular options. If you still don't understand or agree, let your doctor know right away, so he can alter your treatment plan to better accommodate you. Your doctor would prefer to present you with a treatment plan that you will follow, than to issue one and find out weeks later that you did not follow through with it. If you cannot reach an agreement on your treatment, you have the option of finding a new doctor for a second opinion. The choice is always up to you.

When discussing treatment with your doctor, there are several points that should be covered. Exercise 12-2 lists several questions that you might wish to discuss with your doctor. In the next few pages, we will elaborate on some of these questions to give you a better understanding of the type of information you should expect from your doctor.

....
It is important that your treatment plan is realistic for you; one that you will follow.

WILL YOU FOLLOW THE TREATMENT PLAN?

As we've mentioned earlier, a major issue today in medicine is non-compliance. This means that patients do not follow their treatment as prescribed. This may be in the form of only taking half of the prescription, of not doing the prescribed exercises, or not going for a recommended consultation. After you have discussed the questions in Exercise 12-2 with your doctor, you should know if you can and will comply with treatment. Please don't kid yourself. Your intentions may be good, but how is your follow through?

It is very easy to start out "gung ho" only to have indifference replace enthusiasm. Whatever the reason, for any treatment plan to work, you have to follow through. You are more likely to follow through on the treatment plan when it is practical for your lifestyle and when you understand why each aspect of your treatment plan is necessary. If you realize that you will not likely follow through with the treatment plan, then tell your doctor and start a new treatment plan that can work for you. Understanding the WHY of treatment can be an important motivator. This is especially true for complex or painful aspects of a treatment.

HOW DOES YOUR DOCTOR FOLLOW-UP WITH THE TREATMENT?

All treatment plans have a beginning, of course, but they may not have an end. Many conditions are controlled but not cured. If your condition is chronic, then you should receive instructions concerning the appropriate time for you to follow-up with your doctor. At the follow-up, additional testing may be needed and your treatment plan revised. In fact, the whole process might start again.

HOW LONG BEFORE YOU IMPROVE?

Some treatments work rapidly whereas others may take months to exert their full therapeutic effect. Your doctor should provide an estimated time regarding your treatment. It's much easier to be patient and wait for improvement if you know that it may take a few months. However, if a treatment is expected to work rapidly but doesn't, you should consult your doctor in order to review your diagnosis and treatment plan. If your condition begins to worsen rather than improve, you should definitely consult your doctor sooner rather than later.

During the treatment your symptoms may become worse or change before they improve, so again, it is best to find out from your doctor what to expect. Finally, if improvement occurs, whether it is slow or dramatic, a call to your physician may not be necessary but would be a nice gesture to let her know that you are doing well.

ONE THERAPY OR MULTIPLE THERAPIES?

Is your treatment simple or complex? Are you going to have to take one drug or many? Are you going to have to combine drugs and physical therapy? Have surgery? Understanding these and other questions regarding combinations of therapies will help you to schedule your time and make the necessary adjustments to your day-to-day living.

WERE YOU GIVEN OPTIONAL THERAPIES?

Think of your doctor as a waiter. He will give you a menu with choices and, perhaps, even recommend a house specialty. You are free to choose among those listed, or maybe even request something not seen on the menu. If you don't find a dish to your liking, you may want to look at the list once again or perhaps think about going to a different restaurant.

It would be rare for only one treatment to be available for a given problem. Even strep throat has numerous antibiotic choices. Angina (chest pain) can be treated with several types of medication as well as surgery. A ruptured disk in your back can be treated with physical therapy, injection therapy, chiropractic care, medications, surgery, or even without active therapy—letting time heal the back. Choosing a particular therapy is often more challenging than finding one. That is why it is important to ask about alternatives.

IS THIS TREATMENT ROUTINE, UNUSUAL, OR EXPERIMENTAL?

ROUTINE TREATMENTS are tried and true standards. They are the classics (the golden oldies) that most practitioners would use and recommend. For example, insulin injections for diabetes, penicillin for strep throat, and surgery for appendicitis.

WHAT WOULD CONSTITUTE UNUSUAL? One person's unusual may be another's routine. Generally speaking, an unusual treatment would be used by only some physicians while others would be skeptical of its benefits. But remember, this is relative. To traditional physicians, naturopathic cures may seem unusual and vice versa.

TODAY'S EXPERIMENTAL TREATMENTS may become tomorrow's standards. Just look at bone marrow transplants, which were once experimental but now commonplace. Experimental treatments go beyond "unusual" in that they use medications, surgical techniques, or other therapies that are only available through supervised research protocols. The entrance requirements into these experiments are strictly controlled. Also, the research is closely monitored by an investigational review board (see page 293), as is the research team conducting the tests and the organization that is sponsoring the research. One should thoughtfully weigh a decision to participate in any experimental treatment. There are often unknown elements which may expose you to some risk. Plus, you possibly may not benefit from the therapy. The choice is entirely up to you.

If your doctor does recommend unusual or experimental treatment, you should ask for all the literature available on the treatment, so that you can make an informed decision. As part of your request, see if you can get some data comparing the results and outcomes of the experimental treatment to the traditional treatments.

If we choose to stretch the word experimental, medications not formally approved for particular uses by the FDA might be considered experimental. A drug can be used by a physician for any disease at her discretion. If a drug has approval for use for one disease, it then may become widely available for use with other diseases. For example, cyclosporin is a drug used in organ transplantation. It has also been used to treat Crohn's disease and lupus, even though it is not expressly approved for these diseases. Insurance companies may not acknowledge this stretched definition and classify the alternate drug uses as experimental to avoid paying for them. As a consumer, you need to be aware of this and consult your insurance company to see if the drugs you are prescribed will be covered under your plan.

All experimental care in hospitals is governed by investigational review boards. But they do not control the care that a doctor may choose to offer in his office. Therefore, patients can be tempted by hyped-up claims of cures that may be exaggerated or false. **When you are assessing experimental and miracle cures, Caveat Emptor–Buyer Beware.**

A SUCKER IS BORN EVERY MINUTE Personalities, even powerful ones, are reshaped by illness. Illness is capable of transforming a cautious and prudent person into a desperate and irrational patient. People pursue treatments that they would have ridiculed when they were well. **The sicker the patient, the more vulnerable the patient.** With each failed treatment, logic wanes until a point is reached when pain and frustration override reason. Under these conditions patients become easy targets for quacks and charlatans. For centuries snakeoil salesmen have preyed upon the enfeebled and the susceptible. By promising miracle cures, vulturous charlatans have stolen whatever fragile strength, hope, or financial resources remain.

To avoid falling victim to medical quackery, we suggest a cautious and thorough investigation whenever dealing with individuals who make claims for cures that embody any of the following characteristics:

The miracle cure that:

1. Promises a safe and easy solution to a difficult and complex problem.
2. Sounds too good to be true.
3. Relies on a secret formula or process that cannot be found in legitimate medical journals or is not approved by the FDA (Food and Drug Administration).
4. Requires payment upfront, even before you have experienced effective treatment and results.
5. Is administered by someone who sounds more like a salesman than a doctor.
6. Is administered by someone who claims to be misunderstood and/or persecuted by the establishment.
7. Is administered by someone who forbids you from seeing other health professionals during treatments.
8. Is administered by someone who lacks credentials that are verifiable through your state or county medical society, professional licensing bureau, or Better Business Bureau.
9. Is not approved by a local IRB Committee (Investigational Review Board).

If you have thoroughly investigated a miracle cure and still wish to participate in the treatment, we advise one last safety check: Go to an independent observer, preferably your primary caregiver or a specialist who you trust and who will respect your opinion, and ask:

• Is there any theoretical validity to the treatment?

• Could the treatment hurt or kill me?

Finally ask, if they will serve as an independent consultant, watching your progress and ensuring that you are not further harmed

This way, if you do get swindled and the treatment turns out to be worthless, you will at least have made your decisions by informed choice.

DO YOU UNDERSTAND THE BENEFITS, RISKS, AND SIDE EFFECTS OF TREATMENT?

Prime No Nocere. First, Do No Harm. (The Fourth Hippocratic Code) Despite all of the major strides made in medicine, physicians still use drugs and treatments that can produce side effects and can cause permanent harm. Physicians ideally should fix problems rather than create new and possibly more serious ones. However, it is often necessary to administer a treatment that has the potential to be worse than the disease. Because of this, treatment options should be presented along with their intended benefits and relative side effects. These side effects should be adequately discussed and you should have a good understanding of them before you agree to treatment.

For example, if your diagnosis is cancer, and your prognosis is poor, meaning you might soon die without therapy, then aggressive toxic treatment would seem reasonable and possibly the only course of action. In this situation, the possibility exists that you might die from the toxic treatment, but without the treatment you most certainly will die. The struggle may be worth it especially if you are cured.

In contrast, high blood pressure usually damages the body slowly, and there are many different types of drugs to control it. If your medication interferes with your thinking so that you cannot function at work or it causes impotence, you should be given other options, including other medications and exercise and diet modifications, in order to minimize any side effects.

Iatrogenic disease is when the physician makes the patient ill usually by prescribing medication or by surgery. In most cases the doctor did not initially make the patient ill. Iatrogenic disease is most often the result of unforeseen or unavoidable circumstances that occur when the physician attempts to cure the patient. An example is the patient (not known to have any allergies) who is given a sulfa drug that causes a severe allergic whole body reaction called Stevens-

Johnson syndrome. This reaction causes blistering and sloughing of the skin (like a burn). If enough of the skin is lost the patient can die. On the other hand, iatrogenic disease can be the result of oversight or even negligence. If this same patient were given a sulfa drug in the future by the same physician this would be a serious error. If Stevens-Johnson syndrome should occur again this would be considered iatrogenic disease caused by the physician's negligence.

INSIDER'S HINT
Answering the question, "Is the cure worse than the disease?" can help you decide whether a given treatment is appropriate for you.

MEDICATIONS

Most treatment plans include medications. Medications are chemicals, natural or synthetic, that are used to alter your body in order to make it function better. For example, if the body accumulates too much fluid, diuretics (water pills) help pump out some of the excess fluid by improving kidney function.

KNOWING WHY YOU NEED A CERTAIN MEDICINE IS A STRONG MOTIVATOR TO CONTINUE TAKING IT. That's why it is important to ask your doctor for a detailed explanation of how a prescribed drug works to correct or combat your disease.

Medication may be administered in many forms. The method and frequency of administration varies depending upon the individual drug and patient-doctor preferences. For example, drugs that are destroyed by the digestive process may require an injection. Listed in Exercise 12-3 are the key questions to consider when a medication is prescribed.

SPECIAL CONCERNS WITH MEDICATIONS

SIDE EFFECTS are the often known but less desirable effects of a drug (this applies to both traditional and natural remedies). For example, anti-inflammatory drugs typically cause stomach upset and, less commonly, diarrhea.

ALLERGIC REACTIONS are a special category of side effects. They are usually unpredictable (for the first event) and typically cause swelling, particularly of the face, rash, and in severe cases, shortness of breath, and abnormally low blood pressure, or death (anaphylactic shock).

DRUG INTERACTIONS are complications that may occur when taking multiple drugs at the same time. These may occur because one drug raises or lowers the level of the other making it either toxic or ineffective. Different drugs may also be toxic to the same organ system. Toxicity may be more than additive (i.e. 1+1=4). For example, anti-inflammatory medication may impair the flow of blood into the kidneys, while a group of medications known as ace inhibitors (used to treat high blood pressure and heart failure) may impair the flow of blood from the kidney. Used individually, there may not be any problems, but when used together, the drugs may cause kidney failure.

It's important to discuss with your doctor possible side effects, allergies, or drug interactions; and even more important, that your doctor knows all the medications that you routinely take—including over-the-counter ones.

MEDICATIONS FROM A DIFFERENT PERSPECTIVE

It should be recognized that:

- Herbs and natural agents are drugs that can heal or create damage. They are often less regulated than FDA-approved medications. What's more, there have been instances where they have been linked to deaths (tryptophan- and ephedrine-related deaths).
- Foods can be considered and used like medications. Caffeine in coffee, tea, and chocolate, for instance, has been used for generations to self medicate and stimulate individuals (the morning cup of java). Functional foods (also known as *nutraceuticals* or *foodaceuticals)* are also being developed that have special health benefits. Diet can be used to regulate mood through control of blood sugar. It can also control atherosclerosis, blood pressure, and other health functions. Books like *Enter the Zone* by Barry Sears discuss how balancing fat, protein, and carbohydrate intake may be used to optimize body functions.
- Medications can be viewed as controlling basic body chemistry rather than being used for a specific medical indication. For instance, serotonin reuptake drugs were initially used to treat depression but can be used for many other functions, often in lower and safer doses, to treat conditions such as over eating, sexual dysfunction, and premenstrual syndrome (PMS).

Finally, health food supplements such as melatonin (utilized for improving sleep) may prove useful in improving body functions. However, we caution against overuse and abuse of these FAD super hormone and boutique supplements. Their effects are unknown long term. They are FAD not FDA solutions.

INSIDER'S HINT

Be cautious when considering FAD solutions.

THOUGHTS, HABITS, AND LIFE CHANGES

Just as medications can change your health, so too can your thoughts and habits. In fact, it has been said that by changing your thoughts you can change your habits. And by changing your habits you can change your life. Better dietary habits, exercise, and improved sleep are the cornerstones to wellness. Decreasing anxiety and improving mood through laughter, more sunshine, and exercise, plus changing food habits may provide some of the strongest long-term health benefits. Natural solutions for improving mood are discussed in *Beyond Prozac* by Michael Norden. Hundreds of books have been written on dietary habits. Dean Ornish has written several books, including Dr. Dean Ornish's *Program for Reversing Heart Disease,* which discusses a low-fat approach to diet. The book *Enter the Zone* by Barry Sears is a current and thoughtful but still controversial presentation of changing body chemistry through food, which discusses a more balanced approach to diet. It has spawned the *30-30-40* craze. The best solutions for improving sleep probably lie in good diet, exercise, and diminishing psychological stress. And *Power Sleep* by James Maas is a newly published approach to sleep.

In books such as *Anatomy of an Illness* by Norman Cousins and *Love is Letting Go of Fear* by Gerald Jampolsky, the effectiveness of reducing stress and increasing positive body chemistry is discussed. In the book *Personal Power* by Anthony Robbins (also available in cassette tapes, which many feel are a more effective resource), methods are outlined for creating a change in behavior using neuro-linguistic conditioning, a method touted for reprogramming your brain much like you reprogram a computer. Viktor E. Frankl, in *Man's Search for Meaning,* explores the attributes found in survivors.

SURGERY AND INVASIVE/INTERVENTIONAL PROCEDURES

Many treatment plans include surgery and interventional procedures. As a general rule, "less is better." If there is an alternative to surgery, explore that option. If the alternative is appropriate for you than you may wish to attempt that first. However, it is imperative that you:

- Avoid turning an elective procedure into an emergency procedure.
- Do not procrastinate if it is determined that you require surgery, especially if there is the possibility that delaying care could transform a curable condition into an incurable condition.

Emergency procedures almost always carry a higher complication (morbidity) and death (mortality) rate. To decide what is appropriate you will need to rely on the judgment of your doctors (first and second opinion). If you must undergo surgery, ask if "mini" surgeries such as laparoscopic and micro surgical procedures are applicable to your condition.

Some diseases once treated by surgeons are now cared for by non-surgical specialists including cardiologists, and interventional and oncologic radiologists. Radiologic procedures are called percutaneous procedures, meaning the entire procedure is performed through a needle and/or a catheter (plastic tube) that is inserted through the skin. Biopsies, angioplasty (treatment of clogged arteries using balloon), and even treatment of prostate cancer (seed implantation) are just some of the procedures that can now be performed percutaneously. In general:

Most Invasive: Full Surgery
Less Invasive: Laparoscopic, Mini and Microsurgery
Least Invasive: Percutaneous Procedures

OUTPATIENT OR INPATIENT TREATMENT?

As with testing, most treatments are administered on an outpatient basis. Inpatient treatments are required if monitoring is needed or if you are sick enough to require hospitalization. Even complicated chemotherapy is now routinely done on an outpatient basis as are relatively uncomplicated surgeries. However, if you need medications that are routinely administered in a hospital or by a trained medical professional, discuss with your doctor the possibility of using a home nursing service to administer the medications. There may be advantages to having your treatment performed on an outpatient basis. Knowing that you will be able to receive your treatment and go home to your own bed to recuperate can often make you feel better and heal sooner. However, if you feel that you need to stay longer in the hospital make that known to your doctor.

LEARNING MORE ABOUT MEDICATIONS, SURGERY, AND OTHER PROCEDURES

Several sources provide information about medications—their mechanisms, effects, and complications. *The Physician's Desk Reference* is a comprehensive reference book listing prescription medications. It lists the package insert material that has been approved by the FDA. *Facts and Comparisons* is another reference book and it can usually be found at pharmacies or hospitals. Most pharmacists also subscribe to computer information services that can print out information about your medications and interactions.

To learn more about a particular surgery or invasive procedure and its alternatives it is best to ask your physician or obtain a second opinion. For technical details and/or a comprehensive discussion of complications you can read one of the medical-surgical textbooks that is written for doctors. These can be obtained through the local library. Examples of these include *Harrison's Principles of Internal Medicine* edited by Anthony Fauci and *Principles of Surgery* edited by Seymour I. Schwartz, M.D. Other sources of information include the *Consumer's Medical Desk Reference* by Charles Inlander which is a comprehensive medical care reference; *The Cancer Survivor's Almanac* by the National Coalition for Cancer Survivorship which is an excellent reference for cancer patients; and *Prepare for Surgery, Heal Faster* by Peggy Huddleston, which is a five-step mind-body approach to enhancing healing and recovery from surgery. The book *Alternative and Conventional Treatments* by Time Life is a current publication written for the general public. It briefly describes accepted conventional treatments and their alternatives. A complete bibliography of recommended books is listed on page 309.

For information on cutting edge and experimental procedures, you may need to do a literature search on the Internet (see Chapter 4). Of course, an additional way to learn about a procedure and what to expect is to find someone who had that procedure. Your doctor might even provide the name of someone you can call who can answer your questions regarding the advantages and disadvantages of the treatment.

WHAT IF TREATMENT FAILS?

Successful treatment should improve the way you feel. Unfortunately, not all conditions respond to treatment. So what comes next? It's important for you and your doctor to first analyze why treatment didn't work. Perhaps you misunderstood what you needed to do. Maybe other treatments should be considered. Taking more of the exact same medicine may not be the answer. Consider asking for a different treatment plan if the first fails. A second opinion may be helpful for ensuring that the diagnosis and treatment plan is correct. Just remember that finding the treatment that cures or controls your disease may require time.

PROBLEMS WITH THE HEALTH CARE SYSTEM?

Patients need to be aware that doctors today cannot and do not always provide their patients with the best treatment available.

There are three major causes of restricted care:

UNINTENTIONAL RESTRICTIONS. Your doctor may be unaware that there is a better way to diagnose or treat your illness.

BIASED RESTRICTIONS. Your doctor thinks that only he knows what is best for you and denies you access to other treatment options.

INTENTIONAL RESTRICTIONS. Your doctor may be pressured into restricting your care by his organization or limited by your insurance coverage.

CATEGORIES OF SUB-OPTIMAL CARE

FAILURE TO USE THE BEST MEDICATIONS *Example:* The best treatment for your ulcer is a new generation medication because it is more effective and has less side effects. But it is not covered by your insurance. As a result your doctor prescribes and treats you with the older, generic medication because it is cheaper. Unfortunately, it does not solve your problem and you suffer from several side effects. No one tells you there is a better treatment that could treat your ulcer more effectively and without side effects.

FAILURE TO PERFORM THE BEST TESTS *Example:* You are suffering with knee pain and suspected torn cartilage in your knee. Your doctor recommends an arthrogram (injecting contrast into the joint) not an MRI. No one tells you that there is a non-invasive test (an MRI) that can provide an accurate diagnosis painlessly.

FAILURE TO REFER OR PROVIDE SECOND OPINIONS *Example:* You are having unexplained rash, daily fevers, and joint pain. Your doctor's diagnosis is menopause, stress, and degenerative bone disease. Hardly any testing is performed and you ask for a second opinion. But she feels it is unnecessary and denies your request. No one tells you that there are infections (such as tick bites) that can cause this problem and can be diagnosed with a blood test and easily treated with antibiotics.

FAILURE TO OFFER THE CORRECT TREATMENT *Example:* You have unrelenting back pain that shoots down your leg. It causes you to lose the job you love. You refuse to take narcotic medications, and instead suffer with the pain which is taking its toll daily. No one tells you there are treatments less severe than surgery which may give you relief. These include regular physical therapy session, injections of steroids and novacaine-like medications, acupuncture, ultrasound, and electrical stimulating devises.

FAILURE TO TAKE THE TIME TO LISTEN *Example:* Your teenager has a serious behavioral problem that is disrupting the family. The pediatrician just doesn't have enough office time to sit down and fully explore the problem because his HMO has told him follow-up visits can last no longer than 10 or 15 minutes. He is rushed and would like to take the time but feels too pressured to give you the time you need. He suggests a referral to a psychiatrist, which your child refuses (your teenager would sit with the pediatrician whom she trusts). No one tells you that you can write to the HMO Grievance Committee and request strongly that your pediatrician be given enough time to counsel your family.

FAILURE TO SUPPORT PREVENTION *Example:* Your family has a strong history of breast cancer or prostate cancer. Your managed care insurance does not pay for mammograms or PSA levels before age 50. No one tells you that you can petition the managed care program for the test. If this request is denied, you can have a lawyer in a letter strongly encourage that the test be performed, explaining that they will be held responsible for any complication that might occur because of a failure to diagnose the condition.

These and other examples of sub-optimal care support the need to be a proactive patient. Chapters 14 and 15, in particular, provide insights and strategies for receiving the care you deserve.

HEALING

Grace had fought her breast cancer with chemotherapy, surgery, radiation, prayer, faith, and laughter, which helped her survive two precious years longer than anyone predicted. But now it was time for good-byes. She even told her husband to remarry and that as soon as she reached heaven she would search Seattle to find the right women to send to him. As she lay in her hospital bed, her husband crawled under the covers and held her as she took her final breath. Grace's nurturing spirit had been the cornerstone of her life. It is what helped her to battle cancer, and it is what made all the moments of her life, especially the final ones, precious.

HEALING MEANS BECOMING WHOLE AGAIN

With a minor illness, healing may require a handful of pills or an ACE bandage to achieve a complete recovery. But if an illness is more severe, it can tear into the fabric of your life, damaging your body and mind. Healing a serious illness requires much more than pills and potions. It means becoming whole again—physically, spiritually, and emotionally.

The word *healing* originates from the old English word *hal*, which means whole. And when facing a severe illness, each individual must find his or her own unique way of becoming whole again.

When illness alters the flow of life, the mind and the body have the power to adapt. As with many challenges, though, our ability to adapt depends on how we respond to illness often more than the illness itself.

Take Tom, for instance. When he was young he had both legs amputated after a car accident. Not long after, though, he decided that he wanted to run the 50-yard dash again. Sure enough, with the aid of two prosthetic legs that he helped develop, he learned to walk and then to run. Michael, on the other hand, suffered a low back injury that caused intermittent but controllable pain. Still, it forced him to give up the competitive amateur basketball he loved. He went on disability, and soon became depressed, turning to alcohol and seemingly giving up on life.

On the surface, these two stories and their outcome make little sense. Tom, who had greater physical challenges triumphed while Michael was defeated. Both suffered a physical wound, but the man who was defeated by life also suffered a spiritual wound. Tom chose to persevere until he was victorious; Michael became a victim. These two stories reveal that what shapes our lives is not as much the events that happen to us as it is our response to those events. What ultimately determines our triumphs and defeats is our will power, our response, and the meaning we give to the events of our life.

Illness may at first create anxiety, fear, and a sense of loss. Initially you may feel only pain or fear. Rather than running away from that fear, face it. Embrace your fear and become its master. Those individuals who are able to persevere through this challenging period of fear are usually rewarded with a new equilibrium, a sense of well-being and feeling of again being whole—albeit a different whole.

Illness and the process of healing commonly produce new insights. And for some people, these insights are so profound that an epiphany or a metamorphosis occurs in which core values, beliefs, and rules are rebuilt, rebalanced, and redefined. For those individuals, the meaning of their illness is not a curse but a blessing.

INSIDER'S HINT
....

Embrace your fear and become its master.

THE PERIOD OF ILLNESS AND HEALING CAN BE USED AS A TIME TO REINVENT YOURSELF. If you can no longer ski, consider taking up swimming or hiking. If surgery leaves you feeling physically inadequate, such as after a mastectomy, consider the idea of reconstructive surgery. Equally and probably more importantly, consider changing your focus. By exploring the unexplored parts of yourself, you may discover new ways of expressing, feeling, and receiving love and intimacy.

YOU MAY HAVE TO GIVE UP SOMETHING TO GET TO THE NEXT LEVEL. Healing demands a shift in points of view. Most commonly this shift is out of the physical and into the emotional and spiritual aspects of life. As physical power wanes with age or illness, emotional and spiritual awareness may be strengthened. Similar to the blind person whose sense of smell and hearing compensate for the loss of vision, the body that is less mobile and agile can find new freedoms and fulfillments in reading, writing, meditation and painting when it opens the mind to adventures dormant or previously unexplored.

If illness is severe enough to rob the body and mind of self, then death may be the final healing and freeing process. As is sometimes the case with Parkinson's and Alzheimer's disease or cancer, the body can lose its ability to compensate or recuperate. The final days before death may be a time of complete loss of self. But the time prior to that loss can be a period of grace and dignity. The power that exists in saying good-bye should not be underestimated. It can be a healing gift to those left behind. Grace knew that.

The memories and teachings of a cherished friend or relative far outlive their natural years. Their love, laughter, wisdom and spirit—their soul and their essence—are carried like seeds into future generations to comfort, serve, and guide those who are left behind. When emotional healing occurs, death merely becomes an end to suffering, not an end to the soul.

CAN ATTITUDE AND FAITH HELP YOUR RECOVERY?

Many diseases are not curable despite considerable advances in basic science and applied technology. To date, cures for the common cold are not available, let alone many forms of cancer. If your options are limited, you and your doctor may need to change the focus of your treatment from cure to working on your acceptance of your condition.

Numerous intangibles affect your health. Do you want to get well? What is your mental attitude? Do you have faith in your doctor, in yourself, or in your God? Positive attitudes, personal faith, and mental well-being clearly affect all the cogs, nuts, and bolts of your "machine." Stress acts as a magnifier of miserableness. For example, research shows that the mortality rate of recently widowed spouses is higher than that of other people their age. Some researchers have also suggested that prayer may create a better chance of getting better. It isn't quite scientific yet, but most doctors would agree that a patient's personal belief in getting better increases their chance of improving. Thoughts and faith do influence biochemistry.

DON'T LET ANYONE STEAL YOUR FAITH

Mrs. Chen's husband had suffered a severe brain stroke that left him in a coma. The doctors offered little hope for recovery. Yet Mrs. Chen saw improvements in her husband. Over the month he had begun responding to commands and acknowledging her presence. To her this was real progress. To the doctors it was too little too late.

As a result the doctors reported to her that there was no progress to be seen. But their words contradicted her observations, so she lost trust in her doctors. She couldn't help but wonder why they remained so negative when she observed at least some encouraging signs of improvement.

One day she asked one of the doctors why they downplayed Mr. Chen's progress. He explained that because the stroke had been so serious, they didn't want to create a false sense of hope. Mrs. Chen responded that she understood the seriousness of the situation, but questioned why the doctors couldn't at least acknowledge that her husband had made some unexpected progress. "You need some hope to enter the room every day," she said. "Why do you take that hope away from me?" The doctors' attempts to be realistic were stealing her hope.

INSIDER'S HINT
If a doctor is stealing your hope, explain to him what his behavior is doing to you and your family.

THE PLACEBO EFFECT: THE SCIENTIFIC MEASURE OF FAITH

A placebo effect is the body's positive response to a treatment that is *medically* ineffective. The term *placebo* came from the mistranslation of the 116th Psalm in the Hebrew bible. "Placebo" (I shall please). Later, placebo came to mean "make-believe." But the biochemical effect of placebo is far from make believe. In fact, the placebo effect is quite powerful.

If you expect a certain outcome, your body can release chemicals to produce that outcome. For example, if in an experiment, a group of people receive a powder blue sugar pill but they are told it is a tranquilizer, a significant number of individuals will behave as if they were on a tranquilizer. This is the placebo effect. It is hypothesized that these people are so convinced that they received a tranquilizer that their bodies produce chemicals which relax the brain. The more the person is convinced that they will be tranquilized the greater the chance they will experience the placebo effect. But placebo only works on some people, and only some of the time.

It is this inconsistency and unpredictability of the placebo effect that makes evaluating new therapies and treatments so difficult. How much of the cure is because of the treatment and how much is secondary to the placebo effect? To answer this question, traditional experiments of a new drug or treatment will include a control group—a group of subjects who are told they are receiving a particular form of treatment, but then do not. For example, a study is performed on people with hypertension. All patients are told they are receiving an antihypertensive medication. Instead of receiving the new hypertensive medication, though, half of the patients receive a sugar pill. The blood pressure of both groups are monitored. At the end of the study the effectiveness of lowering blood pressure is compared between the two groups. In all likelihood, a decrease in blood pressure will be measurable in both the placebo and the new medication group. The effectiveness of the new drug is determined by how well it lowers the blood pressure when compared to the placebo group. This type of study is called a controlled study and it is the foundation of modern western medical research.

One of the major complaints that traditional Western M.D.s (allopathic physicians) have with alternative therapies is that most alternative treatments have not been researched with controlled studies. Therefore it is difficult to determine how much of the cure is placebo and how much is the actual treatment.

The placebo effect accounts for some of the cures and improvements that are observed for both alternative and traditional medicine. This awareness does not negate the effectiveness of a given treatment. After all, it is the positive outcome that counts. If a given treatment gets a high rate of success without serious complications it must be considered an effective treatment even if it is a result of placebo. If used well, the placebo effect can be a powerful healing tool.

HOPE AND FAITH: POWERFUL HEALERS

Like the placebo effect, hope and faith are powerful healing tools. In fact, they are probably all related. By altering your internal biochemistry, your beliefs transform your biology. The word hope takes its origin from the Old English word *hopian,* meaning to expect. Faith is derived from the French word *feith,* meaning faithful. To expect to be healed and to remain faithful to that expectation is a powerful ally and antidote.

Your faith can be in God, in medicine, in your doctor, in self, or in your family. Each of us has belief systems that can both limit and elevate our potential. If limiting beliefs convince you that you cannot be healed, odds are, you cannot. If you have elevating beliefs, these beliefs may be powerful enough to produce curative internal chemicals such as endorphins (to reduce pain), serotonin (to treat depression), or prostaglandins (to improve blood flow).

Healing through faith and willpower are not well understood but have existed throughout time. It is observed that ailing individuals can delay their death until after holidays and special occasions. Doctors observe this phenomenon, but don't know how it happens. Although poorly understood, some mind-body philosophers believe that individuals who have strong healing powers possess some common characteristics. These characteristics include:

- An openness to the miraculous
- An ability to experience healing images, thoughts or feelings
- A strong faith, determination, and/or willpower
- An unwillingness to see setbacks as failures or defeats

Most health professionals have treated at least one patient with strong healing powers whose recovery was difficult to fully explain by pure scientific logic. As a result of these encounters, some doctors employ the strength of the spiritual inner power to heal while others continue to dismiss it. The physicians that dismiss the power of faith may point out that in well-performed controlled studies it has not been possible to conclusively and statistically prove the effectiveness of the power of faith. At the same time, we believe it should be noted that these same studies have not disproved the power of belief on the healing potential.

The effect of a positive, happier outlook on life and a reason to survive (to see a daughter graduate or a son get married, for example) are difficult to quantitate. Perhaps the power of hope and faith should be examined and observed in more of a qualitative than a quantitative manner. Since most western experiments are designed quantitatively, the more subtle positive effects of hope and faith may be overlooked.

All of this leaves the patient and doctor in a sort of cosmic standoff. Even so, knowing faith does little harm and may do some powerful good is a compelling rational incentive for embracing faith and hope as part of the healing process.

INSIDER'S HINT

Faith and hope can serve as a powerful ally in the healing process

Some doctors are leery of giving patients too much hope. They do not want their patients to have false or "magical" beliefs that interfere with needed treatments. Many doctors fear that patients will go into denial and become reckless or short sighted, embracing unproved or unwise treatments that are more hope and hype than substance.

It is important to make the distinction between denial and hope. Denial is based on fear. Hope is based on faith. We do not advocate denial. We are not suggesting that you replace the healing sciences with faith healing. We encourage hope in the face of reality. Some doctors forget that if they fail to give their patients hope, they may likely lose their patients to hopelessness. Faith and science are not mutually exclusive; they are synergistic.

INSIDER'S HINT
....
Denial is based on fear. Hope is based on faith.

Within the mind-body literature is a recurring theme that gives insight into healing—love has the power to heal. We do not wish to imply that everyone will be physically cured by just having faith or being loving, rather we believe that when excellent treatment is combined with a positive emotional state, you will optimize your chance for cure. To understand the power that a positive emotional state has on your physiology we recommend that you try Exercise 12-4.

FINDING A BALANCE BETWEEN REALITY AND HOPE

One of the primary roles of a doctor is to be analytic and have both feet firmly planted in reality. This ensures that treatments are well conceived and expertly administered. Some patients consider this reality-based attitude as being contrary to their well-being. They wish that their doctors would be more encouraging and hopeful. A different way to view this reality-based physician attitude is that it can serve the patient. As long as the doctor takes care of the details, the patient then has the freedom to explore more spiritual approaches.

The doctor and patient are connected in a delicate interplay like a kite and its navigator. If at critical times the string is not pulled taut the kite will crash. Analogously, the string must not be constantly drawn too tightly if it is to reach its full height and potential. The doctor and patient are intimately connected in a similar interchange between the freedoms of hope and the constraints of reality.

WHAT ARE YOUR EXPECTATIONS?

Expectations are important. They are a form of programming of the mind. It is helpful to write out your expectations and discuss them with your doctor and family. Exercise 12-5 will help you focus your expectations. As you explore your expectations, keep in mind the following thoughts:

- Expectations may not seem realistic today. But you are creating a bridge—a series of steps to get you to that reality—you can create empowering expectations.
- Expectations may take the form of more than just recovery of the body. They may include adventures, self-exploration, contribution to others, sharing your love with others, creating beauty in the world, or writing a diary, an article or a book to teach others the lessons you have learned and want to share.

REMEMBER

"...the moment one definitely commits oneself, then Providence moves too. All sorts of things occur to help one that would never otherwise have occurred. A whole stream of events issue from the decision, raising in one's favour all manner of unforeseen incidents and meetings and material assistance which no man could have dreamed would have come his way. Whatever you can do or dream you can, begin it. Boldness has genius, power and magic in it. Begin it now."—Johann Wolfgang von Goethe

INSIDER'S HINT

Your beliefs and expectations can transform your physiology.

Exercise 12-6 on page 207 can be used as a checklist to help you develop your optimal treatment formula.

A FINAL WORD

Believing you can be cured may not cure you if you are incurable. But what if your chance for a cure is precariously balanced on that mythical scale, with recovery on one side and illness on the other? Could developing a positive healing attitude produce enough potent recuperative chemicals and defenses within your body to tip the scales in favor of recovery? Healing beliefs have power. Commit, believe, and expect yourself to heal.

Treatment Response

1. Please rate your level of pain when you first started treatment, then rate how you feel each week* after treatment. This will help you to determine your comfort/pain response.

    0   1   2   3   4   5   6   7   8   9   10
  Terrible   Poor   Fair   Good   Excellent

2. Please rate your ability to function normally when you first started treatment, then rate your ability to function each week* after treatment. This will help you to determine your functional/dysfunctional response.

    0   1   2   3   4   5   6   7   8   9   10
  Terrible   Poor   Fair   Good   Excellent

3. Please rate your knowledge and application of preventive techniques when you first started treatment, then rate your knowledge and application of preventive techniques each week* after treatment. This will help you to determine your preventive skills.

    0   1   2   3   4   5   6   7   8   9   10
  Terrible   Poor   Fair   Good   Excellent

---

*If you have a chronic or long-standing illness, you may wish to assess your progress on a monthly rather than a weekly basis.

Treatment Plan Questions

These are questions to ask your doctor regarding your treatment plan.

1. What treatment plan do you recommend?

2. Will the recommended treatment require one type of therapy or multiple therapies?

3. What are the alternatives to the recommended treatment?

4. Is the recommended treatment routine, unusual, or experimental?

5. What are the expected benefits, risks, and side effects of the treatment?

6. How long will it likely take before I feel better?

7. Should I call you if I feel worse or better during the course of my treatment?

8. What if the treatment fails or is ineffective?

EXERCISE 12-3

The Medication Questionnaire

Prescription medications can be a great help, that is if they are taken correctly. This exercise covers all the important questions you should ask your doctor when he or she prescribes a new medication.

1. What is the purpose of the medication?_____

_____

_____

2. How do I take it?

    a. How often should I take it?_____

    b. Should I take it as needed or on a regular schedule? _____

    c. Should I take it on a full or empty stomach?_____

    d. What time of day should I take it?_____

    e. How is it to be taken?

    ___ orally   ___ intravenously   ___ other

    ___ intramuscular   ___ transdermal

3. What are the typical or most common side effects?_____

_____

_____

4. If I am taking more than one medication, could there be interactions between the different medications?_____

5. Should I watch out for any food interactions? _____

_____

6. What are the chances that the medication will work?_____

_____

EXERCISE 12-4

The Power of Your Emotional States
(optional but recommended)
This exercise will help you to understand the power that positive emotions such as love and forgiveness have on your physiology. When you perform this exercise feel the change in your body's internal chemistry and ask yourself which is a more optimal state for healing: faith and love or fear and anger? Find a quiet place where you won't be interrupted for 10 minutes.

EXERCISE A: THE POWER OF POSITIVE AND NEGATIVE EMOTIONS
Negative Emotional State Close your eyes. Sit, breathe, and think the thoughts you would if you were depressed. Note your breathing. Is it shallow? Are you hunched over? Do you have a frown?

To Get Out of this State Open your eyes, stand up straight, take a deep breath, clap your hands three times, and scream out a nonsense word quickly *(wob-wob-wob)*. Shake your arms and hands and jump up and down.

Positive Emotional State Close your eyes. Sit, breathe, and think the thoughts you would if you were totally confident and happy. Note your breathing. Is it deep and full? Are you sitting or standing upright? Do you have a big smile on your face?

Concentrate on that feeling, image, and/or sound for one minute while taking deep breaths. While in this excellent state, strengthen this picture of yourself as healthy and vibrant. Feel how good this feels. Say the things you would say to yourself, feeling this great. Make the picture closer and brighter. Make the feelings even more enjoyable and confident. Make the sounds happier and more soothing.

Take a few moments to enjoy this state and these feelings. Then open your eyes.

EXERCISE B: THE DIFFERENCE BETWEEN HOPING AND KNOWING
Close your eyes and imagine how it feels to:
Hope you can pay your bills in the future
Know and expect you can pay your bills in the future (sit up tall and confident and take a deep breath)

EXERCISE 12-4

The Power of Your Emotional States *(cont.)*

Now apply the same principle to getting well. Close your eyes
and imagine how it feels to:

Hope you will get better

Know and expect you will get better (sit up tall and confident
and take a deep breath)

Follow-up Questions As you do these exercises can you feel the difference
in your internal chemistry? Which state do you think would create
a better internal chemistry and frame of mind to optimize your
healing?

In a simple way you have just learned how to change your state
and physiology using your mind. These techniques can be further
developed through yoga, meditation, or neurolinguistics programming. For more information, a list of reference books are provided on
page 310.

EXERCISE C: THE POWER OF MEDITATIVE BREATHING AND IMAGERY (TONGLEN)

Tonglen is a powerful way of dealing with pain, suffering, and loss.
It is derived from a form of Buddhist meditation. This form of meditation works with the power of breathing and positive imagery.

Step 1: Rest your mind. For 1 to 2 seconds still your mind. It should be
clear of all thoughts and in a state of openness.

Step 2: Slowly breathe in the feelings of heaviness, negativity, or dark-
ness that are related to your illness.

Step 3: Slowly breathe out a feeling of lightness, healing, brightness,
and rejuvenation.

Can you feel these qualities moving in and out of your body? Once
you have mastered this feeling, you can work on training your mind to
heal. Whatever occurs in your life, simply breathe in what is not
desired and breathe out what is desirable. Rather than spending your
energy fighting the negative feelings of life, this meditation allows you
to neutralize those negative feelings through the power of breath and
the power of the positive calming of the mind. The scientific explanation for this exercise is that it "tells your brain" you are strong enough
to breathe in the negative, transform it into the positive, and breathe it
out with enough abundance to share your well-being with others.

EXERCISE 12-5

Expectations of Treatment

1. List your expectations of treatment and outcome. Share the list with your doctor, friends and family.

_____

_____

_____

_____

2. Do you believe a positive healing attitude will produce powerful healing chemicals and immune reactions within your body that could facilitate healing?

_____

_____

3. Some expectations for healing may not seem realistic today. But if you can create a bridge, a series of steps to get you to that healing reality, it may be an empowering healing pathway. Write out a step-wise version of how you might imagine helping yourself on this healing path.

_____

_____

_____

_____

4. Expectations may take the form of more than just recovery of the body. What other benefits or positive outcomes do you desire during treatment? They may include adventures, self-exploration, contribution to others, sharing your love with others, creating beauty in the world, or writing a diary, article, or book to teach others the lessons you have learned and want to share. List at least three positive outcomes—besides a cure—that you could begin, which might make a difference in someone's life.

_____

_____

_____

Checklist for the Optimal Treatment Formula

1. Ensure that you have the correct diagnosis.

2. Know your desired outcome and treatment expectations.

3. Develop an effective and achievable treatment plan. Divide it into practical stages.

4. Develop a positive healing attitude
   • Know the positive outcome you desire at each stage of the healing process.
   • Write down the positive outcome you desire and place it where you can see it daily.

_____

_____

_____

_____

_____

_____

_____

_____

   • Meditate (or daydream) daily about your positive outcome (at least 10 minutes per day).

5. Create greater emotional, spiritual, and physical balance in your life.

6. Follow through on your plan with a positive mental attitude.

7. Continuously monitor your progress.

8. Reevaluate the effectiveness of the treatment plan.

9. Adjust or change the plan and expectations as required.

10. Talk to people with your medical problem who have been cured, and consider copying some or all of their behaviors.

11. Implement preventive measures to strengthen the body and avoid recurrence.

Chapter 13

Prognosis

John was 45 when he had his first heart attack. His cardiologist was concerned because there was significant damage to his heart muscle. In discussing John's diagnosis and prognosis, the cardiologist felt that because of the damage and the fact that only two of the vessels could be bypassed, John probably had "about 10 good years." John began exercising, eating right, and taking his medicine faithfully.

John had no symptoms until shortly before the 10th anniversary of his heart attack. He began missing doses of his medicine and having the occasional steak and potatoes. His angina (chest pain) recurred. About two months later, John died of his second heart attack. Everyone was shocked because he had been doing so well for so many years. They wondered why after 10 years of excellent health John's treatment became ineffective and his heart failed.

HOW CLEAR IS THE CRYSTAL BALL?

When you are given a diagnosis and immediately ask, "What will happen to me?" you are asking for a *prognosis*—a prediction as to the course and outcome of your disease. This prediction is based on your doctor's knowledge of your disease, taking into consideration any factors specific to you.

Many people press their doctors for a precise and detailed prognosis. They ask questions such as "Will I recover completely?" and "How long will I live?" Attempting to answer these types of questions can be problematic because the same diagnosis has completely different outcomes in different individuals. A prognosis is merely an educated guess.

Doctor's must rely on statistical probabilities generated in clinical studies to predict patient outcomes. They are not soothsayers and they cannot predict the future.

A patient's fate is not cast in stone; it is still a mystery why some individuals quickly succumb to their illness while others have spontaneous cures. It is useful to remember that throughout the various stages of your illness your outlook may appear to change more than once. Therefore, especially early in your illness, it is helpful to consider your prognosis a "best guess," a work in progress with the final prognosis still to be revealed.

FACTORS THAT CAN INFLUENCE A PROGNOSIS

The type of disease defines the seriousness of your condition. But most illnesses occur as a spectrum of severity. Breast cancer in one person may be slow growing, but in another, it may progress rapidly. Although your doctor can accurately assess the severity of your disease at the time of your diagnosis, he cannot predict how your disease will respond to treatment.

The physical ability of individuals to fight disease varies greatly. The immune system of one person may be able to control a cancer for years or even eradicate it, while the immune system of another may be rapidly overwhelmed such that the person succumbs within a matter of weeks. Your ability to endure the side effects of a prescribed course of drug treatment may also impact the course of the disease. For some people, side effects weaken the body as much as the disease. Your overall physical condition needs to be taken into account when determining the prognosis. Exercise 5-1 on page 71 will help you to define what is normal for you.

The emotional and mental state of a patient impacts outcome. A person who is constantly anxious or depressed may be unable to focus his or her healing energy, thereby jeopardizing the prognosis. People who control their fears are better able to focus on healing, allowing their inner strength to act as an adjunct to their doctor's treatments.

THE ULTIMATE QUESTION: "WHAT IS MY PROGNOSIS?"

There are many crucial moments in your care. One of the most important moments is when the prognosis is discussed. (The manner with which your doctor tells you about your diagnosis and prognosis are important and are discussed in detail in Chapter 11.) When your doctor reveals the diagnosis and prognosis, ask yourself: Does this feel like she is reading a courtroom verdict and sentence or does it sound as if she is preparing me for life's many future possibilities? The difference between these two approaches may have profoundly different outcomes.

A "verdict and sentence" gives most people the sense that their fate is sealed and set in stone. Whereas, a doctor who prepares you for the many possibilities that lie within your future implies a destiny over which you still have some control.

Even for the most critical illness there are options and choices. Do you fight for another day? How do you fight? Can you be at peace with your illness and at the same time use your inner strength and resources to survive? Can you be an example of courage to yourself and your family? These are all choices that you have control over until your last breath.

For less critical illnesses, especially chronic debilitating ones, there are different but equally important questions. How do you learn to live and cope with the loss of normal functions? How can you tolerate pain and overcome disability? How do you approach set-backs and relapses and remain positive in your outlook? Answers to these and many other empowering questions will determine your ultimate happiness, quality of life, and prognosis.

THE BEST- AND WORST-CASE SCENARIOS

Some doctors have a tendency to discuss prognosis in terms of the worst-case scenario. When they do this they are referring to the worst possible outcome for your condition. Some doctors do this so that patients are not unrealistically hopeful or too disappointed, especially if things go badly. If at the beginning of an illness you were led to believe that you would be fully cured, and later you improved but were not as functional as you might have expected, you may become disappointed rather than encouraged by the progress. Perhaps a better approach than the worse-case scenario is a balanced approach. This is where you:

- Are aware of the worst-case scenario and can prepare yourself in a practical manner for its many possibilities, but also;
- Are aware of the best-case scenario where with effective treatment and patient effort you can hope for the best probable outcome.

By knowing the best-case scenario, your brain (which is a powerful computer) is given the opportunity to figure out what strategies to use for achieving some if not all of the desired best-case outcomes. Once your treatment has begun you can then measure your progress on both a daily basis as well as a periodic (monthly or yearly) basis. By reviewing your progress you can more accurately evaluate your state of health. By adjusting your treatment and attitude, you optimize your care and prognosis. By measuring your progress you also have a better handle on what your future holds. Exercise 13-1 can help you and your doctor with this process.

KEYS TO UNDERSTANDING YOUR PROGNOSIS

Prognosis is a statistical guess. It attempts to predict what will happen to the average person given the same circumstances and illness. In some ways it is like a game of poker. Sometimes the odds are strongly in your favor yet you lose, while at other times the deck is stacked against you yet you win. Few players win attempting to pull a card for an inside straight. Despite this fact, every once in a while someone inexplicably wins against all odds. Perhaps you are that someone. Sometimes the best treatment is a stroke of luck.

Because words are powerful tools in healing, doctors should be cognizant of the message they impart especially when it involves attempting to predict a precise outcome. If your doctor begins to reveal your prognosis as if it is a courtroom sentence, stop her and ask her instead to present your future options in both an encouraging yet realistic manner. Your doctor should know as you do that hope is always possible because there are many unknown factors affecting illness. By applying your skills and the skills of your doctor, together you strongly influence your prognosis.

As an additional word of caution, be aware that what may be good today could be damaging tomorrow. In John's case, he was healthy for 10 years. What caused him do so poorly after that? Could one of the factors leading to John's death have been his doctor's seemingly innocent (and at the time encouraging) declaration that John had "about 10 years more to live"? Did the doctor's words create an internal time bomb that contributed to John's death or was it all just coincidence?

If John had been flexible in his approach and reinterpreted the prognosis presented to him he may have been able to turn what seemed like a limitation into an advantage. Perhaps John could have reinterpreted his doctor's words to mean, "You will live at least 10 years, and considering that you have taken such good care of yourself, you may live even longer!" By creating a positive internal dialogue might John have had the capacity to commute his sentence and prolong his life.

STRIVE FOR OPTIMISTIC REALISM

Consider your doctor's prognosis seriously. But remember your doctor does not have a clear crystal ball. A prognosis is a human being making a "best guess." The only thing certain about that "best guess prognosis" is that there is no certainty.

We encourage something that we call optimistic realism, in which you take into account the beliefs and observations of your doctors, friends, and family so you can prepare for future needs. At the same time, realize that a prognosis is not a verdict, mandate, or proclamation of things to come. It is merely a statistical guess. Your faith, courage, effort, and body's individual response are the most important predictors of your recovery. Exercise 13-2 will help you define your prognosis perspective.

Preparing for Your Prognosis

What are your diagnosis and prognosis?

_____

_____

_____

What is the worst-case scenario (prognosis) for your illness?

_____

_____

_____

What is the best case scenario (prognosis) for your illness?

_____

_____

_____

What prognosis do you believe?

_____

_____

_____

What can you do to influence your prognosis?

_____

_____

_____

Review your progress on a daily basis

_____

_____

_____

What progress have you made?

_____

_____

_____

EXERCISE 13-2

Prognosis Perspectives

A prognosis is not a verdict, mandate, or proclamation of things to come. It is simply a statistical guess. Your faith, courage, effort and body's individual response are the most important predictors of your recovery. Even so, you should be aware of the beliefs of your doctor and family so you can prepare for your future needs. Remember, there is a thin line between hope and denial. If you are facing a serious illness, we encourage proactive optimism (Optimistic Realism).

PHYSICIAN'S PERSPECTIVE

1. Circle the number that best describes your doctor's belief that you have a chance for recovery?

    0   1   2   3   4   5   6   7   8   9   10

No Chance   Average Chance   Excellent Chance

2. How much recovery of normal function and life does your doctor expect?

    0   1   2   3   4   5   6   7   8   9   10

None   Average   All

3. How confident is your doctor about your prognosis?

    0   1   2   3   4   5   6   7   8   9   10

Not Confident   Moderately Confident   Extremely Confident

YOUR PERSPECTIVE

(Consider asking family members to answer these questions about you.)

1. Circle the number that best describes your belief that you have a chance for recovery?

    0   1   2   3   4   5   6   7   8   9   10

No Chance   Average Chance   Excellent Chance

2. How much recovery of normal function and life can you expect?

    0   1   2   3   4   5   6   7   8   9   10

None   Average   All

3. How confident are you about your prognosis?

    0   1   2   3   4   5   6   7   8   9   10

Not Confident   Moderately Confident   Extremely Confident

Chapter 14

The Changing World of Medical Insurance and Health Care Delivery Systems

Lolita was tired of struggling to pay her medical bills, and she was too embarrassed to ask for help and doses that were needed to keep her transplanted heart beating. She began skipping doses to make the prescription last longer. She knew better, but what could she do? As a temporary employee of a large pharmaceutical company she received no medical benefits. She made too much money to be eligible for public assistance, but not enough to pay for all the anti-rejection medications and treatments that had kept her alive for 11 years since her transplant at age 13.

The day before her death she called her foster mother and said, "I'm dying. I don't have any feeling in my legs." Her mother replied, "Get somebody to get you to the hospital." Lolita responded, "I don't want to bother anybody."

Lolita was seen by a doctor but it was too late. Before she died, she related, "I just got tired of fighting for medicine, tired of bills—just tired."

Lolita's story, which appeared in a 1995 Associated Press news item, illustrates the problem people with long-term chronic illnesses face: The longer they survive the bigger the medical bills. Lolita was in a Catch-22. To pay for her bills she had to quit college to work. As a result she could not get the kind of job that provided health benefits. Because she worked, she was no longer eligible for full public assistance.

More than ever, having insurance and choosing the right insurance program and health care delivery system can be a matter of life and death. Therefore it is imperative that you choose wisely. It starts with knowing and understanding what you are getting out of your insurance. This chapter is intended to familiarize you with the different health care insurance programs available. Chapter 16 will guide you through the process of choosing a health care insurance policy.

THE EVOLUTION OF MEDICAL INSURANCE

For most purchases, we shop around searching to find the best product, with the best quality, at the best price. And when we find it, we pay for it directly. This is rarely the case in medicine. Often we are sent to a doctor who we know nothing about. We have to trust that this doctor is going to provide us with the best care at a reasonable price. Then when the bill does arrive, we expect it to be completely or nearly completely paid for by our insurance company. If we are asked to contribute significantly to that bill, we often take issue with the request for payment. Frequently, the doctor has no idea what he charged for his services. Also, the patient often has no idea how much the insurance company reimbursed the doctor. This whole process leads to a sense of disconnection between the doctor, the patient, and the insurance company. Have you ever wondered how we got from reimbursing our physicians directly to this complex insurance system?

Ancient civilizations valued the art of healing and often considered it a priestly endeavor. Shamans were honored as tribal leaders. Roman physician slaves were repaid with freedom, if they saved their master's life. In Mesopotamia, the "Code of Hammurabi" describes exorbitant fees for successful medical service. "If a doctor has treated a freeman for a severe wound and cured the freeman…then he shall receive ten Shekels of silver." (Ten shekels of silver was two years' mortgage for a middle class dwelling.)

In the middle ages, kings and land barons managed and rationed out care to the peasants under their control. The land barons determined what care the peasants could receive and would directly compensate the physician for that care. After the middle ages, medical guilds formed. Physicians divided themselves into surgeons and medical practitioners, beginning the era of specialization. Also, much like any other craft, medical charges became standardized by these guilds. Unfortunately, there was little standardization of the medical skills or training.

During the 18th and 19th centuries, the practice of medicine in the eyes of the public was so abysmal that medicine was not only considered useless, it was considered harmful. In 1910, a report titled, "Medical Education in the United States and Canada," brought to light the fact that there were no standards of academic training for doctors, and most doctors learned their trade from influential practitioners and not from universities.

The outcome of this report was the creation of the medical degree and medical schools accredited by the American Medical Association. This in turn generated a great exchange of information which led to new procedures and discoveries. Shortly after the Great Depression, antibiotics, steroids, antiseptic surgery, and improved anesthesia provided a new confidence in doctors which in turn resulted in escalating demands for medical care. As the quality of the medical profession improved, the cost of providing care grew rapidly.

Both before and during the Great Depression, the financial arrangements between patient and treating physician were personal. Patients paid what they could, when they could. Baked goods and chickens were exchanged for health care. In most communities, the bonds between patient and doctor were not only financial but personal.

As the Great Depression and World War II approached, medicine grew more sophisticated and specialized. A more reliable, standardized, and impersonal method for reimbursing physician services was required. It was during Franklin D. Roosevelt's presidency that medical health insurance took root. The goal was to ensure each American affordable health care and provide hospitals and doctors with guaranteed reimbursements.

In 1934, in response to these socioeconomic changes in medicine, independent state insurance plans were united into the Blue Cross Plan. In 1939, the California Medical Society created a Blue Shield Plan to pay physicians' bills in hospitals. With the inception of these two fee-for-service programs, private pay medical insurance was up and running. Fee-for-service medical insurance reigned through the 1980s.

Nowadays, there are many ways to pay for health care including fee-for-service, capitated health plans, workers' compensation, Medicare, Medicaid, and other newly emerging payment methods. From humble patient/doctor transactions, health insurance has grown into a multi-billion dollar multifaceted industry.

Not many people see the business side of medicine because they interact financially with the insurance company and not the doctor.

Unfortunately, doctors also rarely know the true cost of the care that they are delivering because of the negotiated fee schedules they arrange with insurance companies. The health insurance industry has weakened the patient/doctor relationship. Put simply, medicine has become the business of insurance companies. The insurance company's role is now as important if not more important than the doctor's in determining your level of care. That is why it is so important for you to fully understand your health insurance.

TYPES OF HEALTH INSURANCE
Health care insurance can be divided into two categories: private pay and government sponsored health insurance.

PRIVATE PAY HEALTH INSURANCE
Today, most individuals acquire their health insurance through private or publicly owned insurance companies. These companies are usually in business to make a profit for either the private owners or the stockholders. These companies typically offer a wide range of policies, thus coverage will vary greatly between them. The companies usually offer coverage to both individuals and groups. The only outside regulation of these companies comes from the individual state insurance commissions and the Securities and Exchange Commission, if the company is publicly owned. There are three forms of private pay health insurance available to consumers:
1. Not-for-profit plans
2. Other commercial plans
3. Capitated plans

Not-for-profit plans include plans such as Blue Cross and Blue Shield. Other commercial plans include companies that sell insurance to make a profit, such as Metropolitan. Capitated plans are most commonly associated with health maintenance organizations such as Kaiser Permamente.

GOVERNMENT SPONSORED HEALTH INSURANCE
There are three forms of social health insurance in the United States today. The specifics of which will be discussed later in this chapter.
1. Workers' compensation
2. Medicare
3. Medicaid

How Do Health Insurance Plans Work?

Today's health insurance industry is quite complicated. There are many variations in the private pay health insurance practices along with many rules used by the government sponsored programs. Additionally, there are different ways in which you the consumer pays for health insurance and several ways in which the insurance companies can control the delivery of health care.

How Providers are Paid

The most familiar form of physician payment is fee-for-service, commonly associated with private pay health insurance. Fee-for-service was created with the inception of the Blue Cross and Blue Shield Plans. Under fee-for-service, you or your employer voluntarily contract with an insurance carrier to cover your health care costs. A regular monthly premium is paid to the insurance carrier who in return agrees to provide financial reimbursement or compensation to your doctor for your medical care.

With fee-for-service insurance, you decide which doctor you want to see and when you want to see him. The doctor submits a bill for his services to the insurance company and the insurer then pays a portion or all of the bill. The balance of the bill, the portion not covered by the insurance company, must be paid by you.

The other form of physician payment is capitated payment, commonly associated with prepaid plans. The insurance company pays the provider a fixed monthly fee for each person (enrollee) that has signed up to use the provider. The comprehensive coverage includes all routine medical care as well as preventive maintenance care.

The most prevalent form of capitated payment plan uses an HMO (health maintenance organization) to provide the health care. When you enroll in an HMO you need to designate a primary care provider (PCP). You have the choice of switching your PCP if you are not getting the care that you want, but the choice is limited to the physicians within the HMO. You are also restricted in seeing specialists. Your PCP must pre-authorize any referrals to specialists or the use of specialized tests. For example, if you need a specialist for your migraine headaches, your PCP, not you, decides whether you will see a specialist, whether you can undergo an expensive test, or whether you will receive expensive medication for your migraine headaches.

If you choose to seek care outside of the HMO, you will have to pay for your care entirely out of your own pocket. To accommodate patient needs, however, some HMOs now offer enrollees limited reimbursement and access to physicians outside of the HMO. For this service, the enrollee pays the HMO a premium higher than the standard monthly HMO premium. This hybrid insurance plan is a cross between fee-for-service and capitated coverage and is designed to give the patient greater choice, but at a greater expense to the patient.

WORKERS' COMPENSATION (LABOR AND INDUSTRY; L & I)

In many ways, workers' compensation is a cross between a socially and privately supported insurance company. Employers may or may not choose to insure their workers under the workers' compensation plan. The goal of workers' compensation is to ensure that an injured worker receives quality medical care so that he can return to work as soon as possible. Workers' compensation is administered and underwritten by either a private insurance company, state insurance fund, or a corporate fund. In many ways, workers' compensation has served as the forerunner of the modern managed care programs.

Workers' compensation pays for medically necessary treatment of work-related medical problems. The program administrator determines what treatment is medically necessary. Most usual and customary medical, surgical, chiropractic, and osteopathic services are covered including office visits, diagnostic tests, and treatments. Tests and treatments considered experimental are only covered if the attending physician receives special authorization. The program also provides return-to-work assistance for those workers who need this help to return to their previous job or to a different job.

Additionally, the workers' compensation program provides pensions to injured workers, who because of their injuries are permanently unable to return to work. It also provides pensions to the families of workers who die as a result of work-related injury or disease. The program may also pay for modifications to the work place that allow the injured worker to return to work. To accommodate a disability caused by injury, home and vehicle modifications may be covered.

When injured on the job, the L & I (Labor and Industry) process begins when the worker seeks medical care. The first contact may be with the emergency room physician. After the ER treatment, the worker will be referred to a physician for follow-up care. For less acute injuries, the worker may go to a medical doctor, osteopath, or chiropractor of his own choice. This physician will then be the attending physician. The attending physician's role is to identify the work-related medical problems and to initiate the worker's compensation benefits by filing the Initial Report of Industrial Injury or Occupational Disease.

Evaluation and treatment of conditions pre-existing the industrial injury are not covered by this program. At times there will be a question as to whether or not the condition was the result of a work-related injury or problem. The initial evaluation may be covered until it can be determined whether or not the condition is related to an occupational problem or injury.

Receiving care through Labor and Industry can be very frustrating, especially if you do not get well immediately. Typical frustrations for patients, doctors, and L & I are:

1. Patients who malinger and try to get permanent disability benefits.
2. Patients who have real disease which doctors cannot diagnose and treat effectively.
3. Patients and doctors who agree on a diagnosis and treatment, but then must deal with L & I who refuses to pay for the treatment.

For many workers and doctors, L & I is a bureaucratic nightmare despite how good it may sound on paper.

MEDICARE

During the 1960s, there was a growing burden of escalating medical costs to the elderly and concern that the elderly could not afford and would not receive care. In 1965, Medicare was created under Title 18 of the Social Security act to address these concerns.

Medicare Part A (hospital insurance) provides hospital care benefits, some limited skilled nursing care, rehabilitative services, home health care, and hospice care for the terminally ill. There are extensive rules that list what is covered and what is not under Part A. Part A benefits are paid for out of the Social Health Insurance U.S. Trust Fund.

Medicare Part B (supplementary medical insurance) provides payment for medical and surgical services, diagnostic tests, laboratory services, some other outpatient services, durable medical equipment such as splints and wheelchairs, and a variety of other medical supplies. Part B was designed to complement Part A. Part B coverage requires recipients to pay a monthly premium to the government. Part B benefits are paid for out of the U.S. General Treasury and with private insurance supplements.

Medicare does not cover prescription drugs, preventive services, dental care, hearing aids, eye glasses, or routine checkups or eye exams. Alternative treatments, such as acupuncture, and naturopathic or homeopathic treatments, are also not covered.

From its inception, the federal government through the Health Care Financing Authority (HCFA) has contracted with local insurance carriers to administer Medicare insurance. The insurance company provides the government with a reasonable fee for each medical service. Over time medical fees have been highly regulated to keep down medical costs.

For Part B only, a provider may choose to accept Medicare assignment. Accepting assignment means that the approved charge determined by the Medicare carrier shall be the full charge for the service that is covered. In other words, the doctor agrees to accept as full payment for services the amount the government pays. It is the physician's choice to accept or not accept assignment. Once a year, doctors are asked to sign an agreement with Medicare to accept assignment on all of their patients. If they agree, Medicare pays them a slightly higher rate. Even if a physician doesn't accept assignment on all patients, he may do so on a case by case basis for patients who cannot afford to pay for the non-covered part of their bill. Even with assignment, there is a portion of the bill which is not covered by Medicare. There are 10 different medigap, standard insurance plans (A through J) available and each conforms to federal standards for that particular plan. Managed care insurance companies also provide supplemental Medicare insurance.

MEDICAID
In contrast to social health insurance, welfare medicine is not an entitlement but rather a transfer payment from the government to certain individuals. It is a type of charity. In the U.S., welfare medicine is sponsored and funded by federal, state, and local governments. The federal program, called Medicaid, was created in 1965 under Title xix of the Social Security Act. The federal portion is paid for out of the U.S. General Treasury and the state portions are paid for out of the individual state treasuries. An individual proves eligibility for Medicaid based upon income. Medicaid is primarily

intended for individuals who are receiving cash assistance from the government through either Aid to Families with Dependent Children (AFDC) or Supplemental Security Income (SSI). If you are receiving payment from one of these sources, you are automatically eligible for Medicaid. There are some other categories that qualify you for Medicaid: Children of AFDC and SSI families; 65 and over; blindness; and permanent and total disability.

Hospitalization, office visits, lab and x-rays are covered services. Other ancillary services are limited, such as physical and occupational therapy. Some services, such as mental health and dental, are not usually covered except in an emergency. The states determine how much they will pay for services. As a result of the low reimbursement, physicians may choose not to see patients with Medicaid coverage or limit the number of Medicaid patients they do see. This may limit the choice that a Medicaid patient has in terms of who they can see. Several states are placing Medicaid patients in prepaid HMO plans to help control costs. As with other managed care programs, the PCP determines what services the patient needs. The providers bill the state directly. The providers do not need to get pre-authorization for many procedures and diagnostic tests.

MEDICAL SAVINGS ACCOUNTS

Payments for medical expenses and premium in the past have been almost exclusively made by either the individual, the employer, the government. There is a new program called Medical Savings Accounts. Established under a pilot program, Medical Savings Accounts (MSAs) became effective January 1, 1997. They were created as part of the Internal Revenue Code (IRC) and are similar in nature to IRAs. To qualify for one, you must be employed by a business of 50 or fewer employees or self-employed. Also you must be covered by a high-deductible health insurance policy. This means for an individual policy the deductible must be between $1,500 and $2,250 and for a family policy the deductible must be between $3,000 and $4,500 through 1998. These deductible amounts will be indexed for inflation after 1998. There is also a deductibles test to determine whether your insurance plan qualifies.

Supplemental coverage for disability insurance, dental or vision, long-term care, and medigap coverage will not disqualify you for an MSA. However, you need to be careful if you have multiple coverage under more than one health plan because you may not meet the high-deductibles test. Also, qualified MSA expenditures may not necessarily meet the deductible portion of your health insurance plan. It is to your benefit to fully understand what qualifies and what doesn't under the rules of the IRC and your insurance plan.

Contributions to a MSA are tax deductible in the year that you make them. You may contribute up to 65 percent of the deductible for individuals (up to $1,462) and 75 percent of the deductible for families (up to $3,375). Also like an IRA, you have until April 15 of the following year to make your deductible contribution. Interest income earned on MSAs is treated in a similar manner as interest income on IRAs. As for withdrawals, those for qualified medical expenses are not subject to income taxes. But withdrawals for non-medical purposes will be taxed as ordinary income and subject to a 15 percent penalty if withdrawn before the age of 65.

Since this is a pilot program, only 750,000 MSAs are being allowed annually from 1997 through 2000. The IRS intends to establish cutoff periods throughout the current tax year to control the number of accounts opened. Also it is possible that the MSA program will cease to exist after the year 2000, depending upon the results of the program. Any MSAs created during the pilot program will continue to exist, but if the program ceases no new MSAs will be created after the year 2000.

MSAs certainly provide an opportunity for the individuals who qualify to expand the extent of their medical insurance coverage. However, MSAs also fall under the jurisdiction of our tax laws and as such they are governed by rules and regulations that require a certain level of expertise and understanding. Therefore it is important that you fully understand how MSAs work and consult a tax accountant to make sure that you are properly following the regulations to get the maximum benefit from your MSA without incurring tax penalties.

TYPES OF HEALTH CARE DELIVERY SYSTEMS

The Health Care delivery system you sign up for will define the freedom of choice you will have to determine which doctors and which types of Health Care services you can receive.

There are three types of basic health care delivery categories:
- Completely Open Choice (usually associated with fee-for-service). You have almost complete freedom to choose who and what kind of care you desire.

- Partially Open Choice (usually associated with preferred provider organization programs). You have some freedom but many restrictions on who you can choose and what kind of care you can receive.
- Closed Choice (usually associated with HMOs and managed care programs). You have very limited choice as to who you can choose and what kind of care you can receive.

As a general rule, in health care delivery plans, the freedom to choose is proportionate to premium cost. The less the premium, the less the choice. The greater the premium the greater the choice.

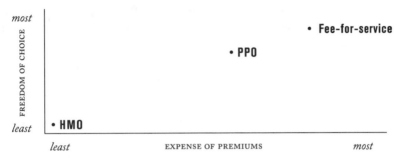

COMPLETELY OPEN CHOICE

This program is usually the most expensive but offers the most freedom of choice. You pay for the care you receive. You can choose almost any doctor or ancillary health care service you desire.

PARTIALLY OPEN CHOICE

This program is usually less expensive than completely open choice programs and offers significant freedom of choice. You can choose almost any doctor or ancillary health care service contracted with your insurance company, within the limits of your policy.

Insurance companies have created preferred provider organizations (PPOs) or preferred provider networks to help control their claim costs and limit patients' access to only doctors who are preapproved by the company. The insurance company selects a panel of physicians to be in the network. These physicians have agreed to accept a reduced reimbursement from the insurance company in exchange for more patient referrals and guaranteed payment. With a PPO plan, when you see a doctor who is on the PPO panel, your bill will be covered at a higher reimbursement percentage than if you get care from a physician who is not a member of the PPO panel.

If the PPO doesn't have the type of doctor you need, then you need to get your doctor to refer you out of the PPO network. If the out-of-network referral is approved by the insurance company, then the insurance company will pay for that service. If the out-of-network referral is not approved by the insurance company, then the insurance company will either reimburse the out-of-network doctor at a lower percentage or not at all. The insurance company does not pay the doctor, and you will be responsible for the entire bill.

It is important to be aware that an insurance company can change its preferred provider list at any time. One year your doctor may be on the list and the next year she may not be on it. This can be either because the doctor has been involuntarily removed by the insurance company or because she no longer chooses to be a member of the PPO.

The advantage of a PPO plan is that you are still operating within a fee-for-service insurance plan. Within the PPO network, you have the freedom to chose the physician and health care facility you believe best meets your needs. An added bonus is that your monthly insurance premiums are typically lower in a PPO than with traditional fee-for-service plans because of the cost savings associated with PPOs.

CLOSED CHOICE
There are variations in how closed your choice may be with an HMO or a managed care program. At the extreme end of the spectrum you may have little to no choice of services and doctors beyond what your primary care doctor and insurance company allow.

INSIDER'S HINT
You always have choice to go outside the limits of your insurance plan at your own expense. Choosing the right policy is crucial.

MANAGING THE DELIVERY OF YOUR CARE
The method by which your care is managed is strongly influenced by both the type of insurance and the type of delivery care system that you have. There are two basic ways of managing your care:
- You direct your own care with the advice and input of your doctor. This is the traditional method by which care was delegated. It is most commonly associated with open and partially open choice programs such as fee for service and PPO plans.

• Your doctor directs your care with advice and input from you. This has existed within HMOs for years, but now this form of management, popularly known as "managed care," has become integrated into other health care delivery systems such as PPOs. It is becoming increasingly important that you understand how it works.

MANAGED CARE

In a managed care plan, you choose or are assigned a primary care physician (PCP) who delivers and coordinates your basic medical needs. Primary care physicians may be prepaid a fixed amount of money per patient on a monthly basis, regardless of the actual services rendered (capitated managed care), or they may be paid on a fee-for-service basis. In capitated systems, your PCP is given a certain amount of money to take care of you no matter how much or how little care he or she delivers to you. Doctors who order too many expensive tests for their patients or give too much care can even lose money. This creates a conflict for the doctor between making money and giving care to the patient.

Because of this management role, the primary care physician is often referred to as a **gatekeeper**. The gatekeeper decides if and when you can see a specialist and what procedures you may or may not receive. For example, in the gatekeeper system, if you have asthma, you cannot see an allergist unless your primary care physician "opens the gate" and makes the referral to the allergist. If your PCP doesn't believe you need to see an allergist, then your insurance company will not pay for you to see one—"the gate is closed."

Because managed care incorporates the philosophy of individual patient case management, it can be used essentially by any type of health organization or insurance plan. The operating principles of managed care are:

1. The gatekeeper should deliver as much medical care as possible (this reduces costs by avoiding more expensive specialists care).
2. The gatekeeper must authorize any referral to any other physicians, such as a specialist or consultant.
3. If the patient goes for consultation or treatment without prior authorization, then the patient is personally responsible for the bill.

4. A consultant cannot order, prescribe, or provide treatment without the approval of the gatekeeper.
5. Care cannot be transferred to a consultant without the prior approval of the gatekeeper.
6. The patient can change gatekeepers, but choice is limited and any change must be done through proper notification of the managed care program.

IS FEE-FOR-SERVICE INSURANCE BECOMING EXTINCT?

Traditional open-choice, fee-for-service insurance is becoming more expensive and therefore less popular, but it is still available. However, since the price of insurance is an overriding factor in determining whether most individuals choose a particular insurance plan, the trend in insurance is to move away from the more expensive fee-for-service policies. Still, there are still some insurance subscribers who place freedom of choice above price.

To entice subscribers who desire choice, insurance companies are becoming more flexible and developing hybrid insurance products such as the HMOs that provide coverage for care outside of the HMO for an additional monthly premium. Insurance companies will continue to offer plans that allow choice only as long as enough patients demand to choose and direct their own health care.

WHO IS REALLY CHOOSING THE HEALTH CARE YOU RECEIVE?

It is important to realize that more than ever, administrators with no or limited specialty medical education are making depersonalized decisions regarding reimbursement for health care. This in turn dictates the type of care that is delivered. The following story illustrates this disturbing trend.

Joe Fender, a metalworker, was scheduled for an MRI scan. In the past, Joe had been treated for injuries to the eye suffered in grinding accidents. Because of this history, the radiologist was concerned that small remnants of metal could still be present within Joe's eye. If there were any shards of metal, they could move during the MRI and possibly cause blindness. To protect Joe from this risk, the radiologist requested a screening CT scan of the eyes to look for metal fragments.

Because the MRI scan was needed to evaluate a work related accident, Joe's referring doctor sent the request for the screening CT scan to the Department of Labor and Industry (L & I). Despite many calls by both the referring doctors and the patient, L & I repeatedly denied the request. Their policy was that they would authorize a two-view x-ray plain film of the eyes, nothing else. L & I insisted that if the policy was not followed, they would send the patient to "Elsewhere General" where the MRI would be performed by just screening plain films. The radiologists explained that the plain film was less sensitive than the CT scan for detecting metal in the eye. And because of this, as a consideration to their patient's safety, the radiologists were routinely performing the screening CT scan for the same price as the screening plain films. Despite this, it still took two hours of the radiologist's time to get the screening CT scan approved. (Of interest, during this same period, an MRI was performed at "Elsewhere General" on a different patient whose eyes were screened with plain film and not a CT scan. That patient suffered damage and partial loss of vision because metal went undetected on plain films. Coincidentally, that was the same hospital that L & I had threatened to send Joe Fender to.)

With all the changes and challenges that medicine is experiencing, it is wise for you to educate yourself so that you can work in concert with your doctor to get the care you need and deserve. These new times necessitate that you become your own best medical advocate. At a minimum, we believe patients should expect and be entitled to the following proposed "Patients' Bill of Rights."

PATIENTS' BILL OF RIGHTS
Patients should...
- Be informed of all their medical options
- Have the right to choose the doctor they want (including specialists) in order to get the care they need
- Have medical decisions made by medical experts not insurance companies, managed care companies, or hospital administrators
- Have access to emergency room care wherever and whenever it is needed
- Have all medical records kept confidential
- Be guaranteed quality care

To guarantee these rights and to get the care you deserve, you will need to:

1. Learn how to communicate effectively with your doctor
2. Get prepared and organized for your appointment
3. Take responsibility for ensuring that you are receiving excellent care
4. Select an insurance plan that meets your medical needs
5. Understand and protect your medical rights

Understanding your medical coverage and choosing insurance wisely is an important aspect of receiving good care.

DETERMINING YOUR PRESENT INSURANCE STATUS

Exercise 14-1 will provide a starting point for evaluating your medical insurance and health care system.

In the next chapter we will discuss the pitfalls of the new managed care style and how to avoid them! And in Chapter 16 we will help you to choose the insurance plan that is best for you.

EXERCISE 14-1

Being Your Own Best Patient Advocate

1. What is your current form of health insurance? _____

_____

_____

_____

_____

2. Are you satisfied with your health insurance? What do you like or dislike about it? _____

_____

_____

3. Do you know how your insurance program evaluates
quality of care?   Y   N

4. Do you know if your insurance plan uses a
gatekeeper system?   Y   N

5. Are you considering changing to a plan with a
gatekeeper?   Y   N

6. If the insurance plan does have a gatekeeper:
   a. Do you know how the gatekeeper is paid? _____

   _____

   b. Do you know if the gatekeepers have financial incentives
      (bonuses) for limiting usage of resources? _____

   _____

   _____

   c. Do you know what happens if the gatekeepers send patients for
      too many referrals or specialized tests? Can they be fired or
      make less money than their colleagues who send fewer referrals
      or order fewer tests? _____

   _____

   _____

7. As a last resort consider getting legal advice.

Chapter 15

Managing with Managed Care

Tom Wilson, an 81-year-old retired CEO, had been in excellent health most of his life until he began experiencing some mild hoarseness and difficulty in swallowing. His doctor, Dr. Phillips, sent him for a CT scan of the throat which revealed a small tumor in the left vocal cord. The radiologist, after identifying the tumor, called Dr. Phillips and informed him of the findings. Instead of asking for details about the tumor, Dr. Phillips asked, "Can you please tell me what insurance this patient has so that I can determine whether I really need to work up his problem?" Surprised, the radiologist asked the doctor why he was so concerned about Mr. Wilson's insurance. "Well, he's very old and an extensive work-up and treatment will be expensive," Dr. Phillips said. "If Mr. Wilson is a member of our managed care program it will be costly to our group. I'm not sure that a work-up and treatment in an 81-year-old is cost effective. After all, this may or may not be cancer."

Stunned, the radiologist responded, "But this is an extremely small lesion which should be completely curable. Whether it is malignant or not, it needs to be treated early. You'd want that type of treatment for yourself wouldn't you?"

At that point, Dr. Phillips was handed Mr. Wilson's chart by one of his assistants. "Oh, there's no problem. Mr. Wilson doesn't have a gatekeeper, and he's not part of our managed care program." Then, in an annoyed tone, he added, "And by the way, you can get off your high horse and holier-than-thou principles. I'll be sending the patient to an ear, nose, and throat specialist without delay."

Mr. Wilson never knew about this discussion. He wasn't aware that his well-being, his quality of life, and possibly his life itself depended on the type of insurance coverage he had.

This story is true. It's a sad example of the changes that are occurring in medicine today. Even sadder, Mr. Wilson's doctor is normally a caring and very competent physician. In years past, this physician would have been focused on the patient's care, not the patient's insurance. The problem today is that doctors like Dr. Phillips are being torn in opposite directions. Doctors are being asked to serve two masters.

TRYING TO SERVE TWO MASTERS

Throughout history the patient/doctor relationship has been a sacred relationship, based on trust. There has been an unwritten contract, a covenant, that the doctor put the patient's welfare and needs above the doctor's material and monetary rewards. This covenant is changing. The sacred patient/doctor relationship is being breached in the Age of Corporate Medicine. Doctors are being asked to balance the needs of patients against the needs of the corporation. Influenced by money and fear, doctors are becoming double agents.

Patients rely on doctors to provide them with the best possible care. But if corporations interfere with the patient/doctor relationship by using incentives or threats, the fabric of the sacred patient/doctor relationship unravels. Mr. Wilson's story is a graphic example of how this conflict of interest now confronts doctors.

INSIDER'S HINT

Doctors should be serving only one master, the patient.

Insurance companies rely on doctors to curb medical spending and limit the use of expensive resources. Doctors once applauded for excellence of care are now applauded for excellence of cost containment. Doctors once financially rewarded for treating patients now receive financial bonuses for not spending money on their patients' health care.

It is easy to be lulled into a false sense of safety because you are under a doctor's care and have health care insurance. However, because the patient's health may no longer be the doctor's only concern, it is now imperative that you **become your own best patient advocate.**

WHY MANAGED CARE? WHY NOW?

The revolution in managed care resulted from rapidly increasing health care costs in the 1970s and '80s. The percentage of our country's spending devoted to health care reached what was felt to be an unacceptable level, and dire predictions of future costs suggested that health care costs would soon bankrupt the country. This was a very real concern.

To better understand the government, corporate, and societal drive to control health care costs, it is important to first ask: What were the factors that were contributing to these escalating costs? And do any of them represent legitimate increased costs as opposed to wasted and overpaid expenses?

Before managed care, two of the dominate forces driving up medical costs were:

- The aging society in which an older population has more illness and requires more care than a younger population and
- New developments in medicine that allowed doctors to diagnose and treat conditions that in the past were not effectively treated.

These new developments—though they may eventually lower the costs of treating a particular disease—prolong life and increase the overall cost of medical care for any given individual. For example, in the past, osteoporosis (brittle bone disease affecting mostly women) was diagnosed when a person experienced a fracture without a significant injury and an x-ray revealed a loss of normal bone calcium density. The problem is, standard x-rays cannot diagnose osteoporosis until it is late in the disease and bone strength is irreversibly lost. Newer methods, such as DEXA (dual energy x-ray absorptometry) scanning can now evaluate bone density with precision before too much damage has occurred. Physicians even now screen women at risk for osteoporosis and start treatments to prevent fractures.

In the past, osteoporosis was treated only with inexpensive medications such as calcium, vitamin D, and estrogen. These medications were cheap but they also were often ineffective. Newer more effective medications, such as alendronate and calcitonin, can reverse bone mineral loss and reduce the risk of fractures. The cost of screening large numbers of people is expensive, and long-term therapy with these medications is expensive. The future benefit of increased quality and longevity of life is often not factored into the health care cost equation. What is the monetary benefit and increased productivity of an individual whose hip fracture is prevented? What is the cost-benefit to the society, the family, and the individual when hip or pelvic fractures are prevented? This osteoporosis scenario is repeated throughout medicine with other diseases such as breast cancer, prostate cancer, and childhood immunizations. The human misery factor and the indirect business savings from preventive care are often not considered or factored into the costs of medicine. If these savings were calculated against the costs of medicine than, medicine might appear less expensive than presently portrayed.

An issue that has rarely been discussed in the same sentence with increasing medical premiums is business savings resulting from preventing illness and treating illness early, rapidly, and effectively. Perhaps it is cost effective for businesses to spend more on prevention and early detection and treatment of their employees. Hidden in the escalating medical costs may be escalating business productivity and profits because their employees are healthier and more vital than they would be if they had restricted access to care. New medications and technology although more expensive, allow workers to stay at work or return to work more quickly than in the past. Is it profitable to a business to have its employees and their families healthy? Is there a monetary and societal benefit of increasing the health standards and the quality of our lives? At the very least, we believe benefits provided by better medical care should receive greater attention and be factored into the cost equation when talking about and estimating the "real" price of medical care. Unfortunately, at present, the only real costs discussed are the expenditure of premiums by employers.

Despite these legitimate expenses and benefits it was felt that medical costs were too high and something had to be done to curb them. Business and government argued that if costs were controlled, more individuals would have access to better and more affordable care.

If you look back 20 years, patients, doctors, insurance companies, businesses, and the government all have had different views of the state of medical care in this country.

Patients, if they could afford insurance, were generally happy because they had nearly complete access to whatever care they felt they needed. They had the freedom to go to any physician, and could direct their medical care. People with inadequate or no insurance, on the other hand, saw medicine as an expensive system that was not accessible. Many individuals viewed health care as a human right that was being denied to them and their family. From these individuals there was a strong outcry to revamp the system in order to create an affordable and accessible health care delivery system.

Doctors enjoyed the freedom to make medical decisions without regard to the cost of those decisions. Many doctors profited handsomely from the tests they ordered or procedures they performed, without having to justify the need or the expense. The more care they delivered the more money they made. Patients also profited because they obtained all the care and tests they required without regard to how much it cost. At times, though, this system was abused by doctors and hospitals in the form of unnecessary surgeries and prolonged hospital stays.

Insurance companies competed for healthy, employed persons, and generally made large profits. But medical insurance premiums were increasing faster than employer profits. And businesses and the government (Medicare and Medicaid) imagined ever increasing expenditures spiraling out of control. Also, expensive new medical technologies (liver and bone marrow transplants) and chronic incurable illnesses (AIDS) were beginning to erode medical insurance company profits.

All of these social circumstances provided the background for the revolution now known as managed care. The current changes in the delivery system are a response to need. The need is that of the patient and the employer to obtain and provide affordable health care.

THE EFFECT OF MANAGED CARE

One of the goals of managed care has been to save money. However, many say it has spawned new problems and new greed from insurance companies, corporations, and managed care executives who see medicine as a pot-of-gold ripe for the taking. A report by the American Medical Association (*AMA News,* April 8, 1996) found "no evidence that managed care, in any form, has reduced the rate of growth of health care expenditures." Much of the money that was once used to treat illnesses is used for expensive advertising budgets and executive salaries and bonuses.

Insurance and managed care companies are in business to make money. The CEOs of large managed health care providers are under intense scrutiny to ensure profits, not lives, for their companies, themselves, and their stockholders. They have received hundreds of millions of dollars in stock options for turning a profit. This massive wealth has been quietly diverted out of the nation's limited health care resources and into the pockets of a few ambitious and clever executives. Billions of dollars that could have made lives more comfortable, saved lives, been used to develop new medical facilities, and fund research have instead been diverted into the bank accounts of a small cadre of individuals who have become wealthy at the expense of those they have been entrusted to cover.

In the past, insurance companies were at risk for rising medical expenditures. However, they have shifted the financial risk from themselves to the physicians and the managed care organizations. In doing so, they have created a conflict of interest for the caregiver—maintain excellent profitability or give care to your patients.

Many doctors see this health care revolution as dangerous. For most including the primary care physician who now has to be a gatekeeper (see page 241), managed care offers less money for patient care, less control over health care delivery, and more paperwork and administrative hassles.

Patients have varied opinions. For some, health insurance is now affordable. They realize traditional health insurance is a luxury, like a Mercedes that most will never own. For many people, though, the change has had a negative impact on their freedom to choose and direct their own health care. They experience frustrations along with their physicians when they cannot get the medicine, the test, the consult, or the procedure they prefer. For them, managed care is involuntary rationed care.

HOW MANAGED CARE PRESENTS A RISK TO YOU

In a way, there has always been managed care. Either your family doctor—or you—managed or coordinated your care. Health maintenance organizations (HMOs) were built on the concept of primary care providers who would coordinate your care. **Unfortunately, to date, managed care has often been more managed than caring.** Patients have become life units. This has further contributed to the depersonalization of medicine. In many instances, physician quality and compassion has become secondary to the effectiveness of a physician to reduce costs. This translates into the doctor being forced to provide less or substandard care. It's an icy compassionless thought, but sometimes a patient's rapid death is more efficient and cheaper than a long, drawn out attempt to save his life.

Physicians are also asked to spend more and more time getting approval for procedures. This takes time away from patient care and continuing medical education. Many physicians have grown weary of battling with insurance companies in order to protect their patient's rights. In simple terms, many physicians have just given up.

MANAGED CARE = RATIONED CARE

Why do physicians have to fight this battle? Managed care operates on the principle that there are limited resources available from which everyone must receive care. Therefore, the services must be prioritized and "rationed out properly." Managed care can be cost effective and may work well for minor illnesses. The problem seems to arise, however, when patients develop more complex illnesses, which require a higher usage of resources. Access to care may be delayed or denied to you because it is considered care of an unnecessary, expensive, or excessive nature. In other words, managed care rations available health care resources.

Instead of being your health care advocate, your doctor has become your gatekeeper rationing out your access to the health care system. Cost control has become a primary gate for your gatekeeper physician who is trying to save more money (or make more money), see more patients, and provide less expensive care on a daily basis.

THE GATEKEEPER The role of the gatekeeper is to coordinate care. This means either permitting or denying access to care. The gatekeeper is a sort of double agent torn between the patient and the corporation, balancing his responsibilities precariously, hoping that neither the patient nor the corporation will feel their trust has been betrayed. By forcing doctors to choose between their patient's health or their corporation's (and often the doctor's) financial health, the doctor-patient relationship is being violated. It is this conflict between money and your health that is pervasive and potentially most dangerous to your health.

PROFILING Profiling is a popular practice of managed care which forces the doctor to serve two masters and encumber the patients' rights. Profiling means the managed care insurance company or HMO monitors how much the doctor spends on tests and treatments. They monitor the length of patient visits. If the gatekeeper spends too much time on you or too much money on your care, then your insurance company loses money. Physicians can lose their jobs in the

HMO/managed care system or lose their preferred provider status in a PPO because of excessive spending. This may be done without concern as to whether or not the spending was necessary or helped patients get better sooner.

Profiles usually concentrate more on cost than quality of care. In fact, doctors who spend less time and money on their patients are often rewarded with the largest financial bonuses. Bonuses are usually given without regard to the quality of care delivered. For example, mothers giving birth were often forced out of the hospital within 24 hours. Doctors who allowed patients to stay for two to three days in order to rest; heal an epesiotomy (surgical procedure performed to enlarge the birth canal); or learn techniques of breast feeding and child care were penalized. It took a federal law to reverse this corporate behavior. It is now legally mandated that new mothers can stay at least 48 hours after delivery.

GAG RULES There are spoken and unspoken "gag" rules from some insurance programs that prevent health care providers from "too fully" informing their patients of their options and rights for care. There is a critical difference between:
- deciding your course of care with your doctor when you have full knowledge of your options;
- deciding your course of care with your doctor when you do not have full knowledge of your options; and
- your doctor deciding your course of care without you knowing.

Patient choice and full disclosure is crucial to adequate medical care.

DISJOINTED MEDICAL CARE Initially, the hope of managed care was that all of your care would go through one individual who could coordinate your care. In part, this has occurred, but unexpectedly, a new form of disjointed or fractured care has developed.

For people who are seen by multiple specialists, there is the trend to have the patient seen as infrequently as possible. This is done to save money. As a result a patient may not receive a routine follow-up visit by her specialist. As a consequence, many interim problems arise that are not detected early by the gatekeeper who is less trained in recognizing and preventing the subtle and early signs of disease progression, recurrence, and treatment complications. The effect is that patients are now managed more by crisis care than by preventive care.

CAVEAT EMPTOR

We believe that how you pay for health care is important. When third party payers (insurance companies) make the payment, the link between patient and physician is weakened. Insurance creates contracts for care between the patient and the insurance company and the insurance company and the doctor. There is no financial link between the patient and the doctor. There is only the moral and humanistic contract between the patient and doctor, which gets overshadowed by the financial contract between the insurance company and the doctor.

We recognize the need for insurance. Insurance is a reality of our complex modern society and it serves a useful purpose. It provides a means for individuals in our society to share risk and thereby acquire affordable health care. However, society needs to find a way for the patient/doctor relationship to have equal footing with the insurance company and doctor financial contract.

We strongly believe that your insurance company should not be making decisions regarding the care and procedures you require. Your doctor is better trained to make medical care judgments than your insurance company.

We strongly believe that your insurance company should not be influencing your physician's decisions by coercion or by incentives to limit treatment. This violates the moral and humanistic contract between you and your doctor.

We caution you against giving up your patient power and surrendering your health care rights to corporate medicine.

BECOMING YOUR OWN BEST PATIENT ADVOCATE

What we are beginning to see in medicine today is alarming, and we caution you to be on the lookout for doctor and corporate misconduct that denies you your right to adequate medical treatment. These warning signs include:

1. Physicians trained in general medicine (but poorly trained in specialized care) attempting to administer complex specialized medical care in order to save money.

2. Physicians not fully informing patients of all the diagnostic and treatment options available. This is often done to avoid having to spend money to treat or diagnose a difficult problem.
3. A delay in care such that by the time the patient is fully aware of the disease, the disease (such as cancer) has progressed and spread so extensively that only the less expensive palliative care (not curative care) is necessary. This is the opposite of preventive care.
4. Insurance companies and managed care companies putting so many obstacles before the patient and the physician that only the most persistent doctors or patients get the care the patient requires.
5. Good and conscientious physicians who are giving up and acquiescing to the pressures of insurance and corporate medicine.
6. Managed care corporations who are black listing, silencing, gagging, firing or denying reimbursement to physicians for giving too much patient care, spending too much money, or speaking to patients about the injustices of their care.
7. Patients receiving fractured care instead of coordinated care. This happens when patients are left to sort through the health care maze on their own instead of receiving the coordinated beginning-to-end care promised by the managed care program.

What can be done to avoid these abuses? You must become **your own best patient advocate.** This requires you to form a renewed partnership with your physician in order to work together proactively, not passively to get the care you need and deserve. It also means that you must form a working relationship with your insurance company and your employer's benefits coordinator. Further, you might need to take action within the community by writing to your local news outlets. You also might need to lobby your state legislator or congressional representative or senator. Exercise 15-1 on page 246 provides a starting point for asking questions about a gatekeeper and managed health delivery program.

MANAGED CARE CAN WORK IF THE DOCTOR SERVES ONLY THE PATIENT

Mary Jane was 21 weeks pregnant. Because of her advanced "maternal age," Dr. Shapiro sent her to have an amniocentesis. During the procedure a tumor was noted in her pelvis. The next day an MRI was performed which defined the tumor's location and provided a differential diagnosis for the mass. The following day the patient had a biopsy that showed the mass to be benign. To the relief of the family the mass was scheduled to be removed after the delivery of the baby.

Dr. Shapiro was Mary Jane's gatekeeper. And Mary Jane was a member of a managed care PPO with a gatekeeper in which there is no capitation. Dr. Shapiro's care was exemplary and no conflict interfered with his doctor-patient responsibility. In fact, he spent more money for Mary Jane's care than the minimum in order to get the care he knew would be the best.

- He sent Mary Jane to the downtown center that specializes in higher risk pregnancies
- He performed an MRI (which is more costly) rather than a CT in order to avoid radiating the fetus
- He sent Mary Jane back to the downtown center that specializes in complicated biopsies

The outcome was a mother and a family that could focus on the delivery of a healthy baby.

Many comments in this section may seem biased against a closed choice health care delivery system and capitated managed care. Quite simply, that is because they lend themselves to conflicts of interest between the patient and doctor. What we hope to communicate is that **we believe in patient choice and in the unencumbered rights of the physician to perform his skills as best as he knows how.** This may be idealistic, but it still should be a goal for any health care system, including closed choice managed care. We believe managed care can only work if patients' rights are respected and doctors serve patients as their primary masters.

Evaluating Managed Care

If your doctor is part of a managed care program, do your best to evaluate the following:

1. Is the managed care program a closed, partially open, or open system? What name does it go by (PPO, HMO, fee-for service)?

_____

_____

_____

2. Is the managed care program capitated? Is the doctor paid a set amount each month to take care of you?

_____

_____

_____

3. If gatekeepers are used, what can you do to get additional care if you disagree with their decisions? What are your rights?

_____

_____

_____

4. Are physicians trained in general medicine and not specialized care attempting to administer complex, specialized medical care in order to save money?

_____

_____

_____

5. Do patients in this program experience significant delays in care? Are they receiving fractured care instead of coordinated care?

_____

_____

_____

Chapter 16

Choosing Your Insurance Coverage

Rolanda couldn't believe it. Her insurance company had canceled coverage for her and her son because their $127.25 insurance payment had failed to include a 94-cent rate increase. The Seattle women was not warned of the cancellation nor was she advised how to appeal it.

Rolanda tried everything she could to correct the situation. But her pleas were ignored. Finally, friends stepped in and called the local newspaper with her story.

When the insurance administrator was asked why Rolanda was not assisted more compassionately before canceling the policy, he indicated that all the needed information was in the insurance manual. He added, "We can't read the benefit booklet to all the people who need that."

It took a while, but when the callous behavior of the insurance carrier was publicized they reversed their decision and reinstated Rolanda's insurance.

START WITH THE FUNDAMENTALS

Feeling personally responsible for another human being's life is a weighty burden and very different from just following orders or making impersonal decisions based on bureaucratic rules. Doctors are trained for years to accept this personal responsibility. On the other hand, insurance companies and their employees are removed from the patient by layers of regulations and bureaucracy. Clerks, often with limited education and no specialty medical education, make depersonalized decisions regarding the reimbursement for health care, which in turn dictates the type of care that is given.

With as many challenges as medicine has experienced it has become necessary for you to become your own best advocate.

Since the best medicine is preventive medicine, the best way to ensure coverage for the care you need is to choose an insurance company that offers and guarantees you the care you may require. Even if your choices are limited or nonexistent, it is important to know and understand what coverage you do have as well as your options. More than ever, insurance coverage may make the difference between health or illness, therefore use your resources wisely. Obtaining the best care you can starts with knowing and understanding what you are choosing.

The task of finding the insurance program that best meets the needs of you or your family can be daunting. Large spreadsheets and tables listing specific benefits and payment options can be as confusing as deciphering Egyptian hieroglyphics. Despite the complexities, it is still important to study the terms and options available with each plan, especially the fine print.

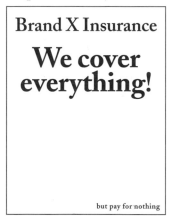

Brand X Insurance

We cover everything!

but pay for nothing

If you are self-employed or if your employer does not provide health insurance, insurance agents can be helpful. Affiliated insurance agents are associated with a particular insurance company. The agent may tell you he chooses not to sell other companies' policies, but the reality is that he is an agent for one or only a limited number of companies. Non-affiliated or independent agents can sell you the insurance policies of many different companies. When using an agent, remember, the choice is yours (not your agent's).

Individual health insurance coverage is purchased directly by individuals for themselves and their dependents. Individual insurance policies generally cost more than group policies because the premium is based upon experience rating. To obtain individual insurance coverage, you will be asked to complete a health history application form and may even be required to have a physical exam. The purpose of this is to determine if pre-existing medical conditions are found. A pre-existing condition is any illness that you have acquired prior to obtaining health insurance. If the insurance company believes that this condition may result in substantial medical costs, benefits for this pre-existing condition may be excluded from the policy; coverage for the existing condition may be delayed for a predetermined waiting period; or premiums for the policy simply may be higher to counteract the expenses the insurance company expects as a result of that pre-existing condition.

Group health insurance is available to a person by virtue of being a member of a particular group, usually an employer or employee group. Group insurance is generally less expensive and easier to obtain than individual coverage. With group insurance, a health history or physical exam is usually not required. Pre-existing conditions may be excluded during a waiting period, usually up to six months, but they will be covered under the same terms as the rest of the insurance contract. In group insurance there are more people assuming the components of the cost and risk for the pre-existing conditions of the group.

How Medical Premiums are Determined

Insurance premiums are determined by two different methods of rating: experience rating and community rating.

Experience rating is based on the actual medical experience of an individual or small group of individuals during prior years. Most insurance policies that pay doctors the typical "fee for service" use experience rating to determine the rates. For instance, if you and the members of your small business have an experience-rated fee for service insurance and no member of your group or their family has been seriously ill, the rates will not rise rapidly. This form of insurance is much like car insurance; the fewer accidents and tickets you have the better your premium.

Community rating is based on the utilization of medical services by a large group or an entire community over a period of time. Most managed care programs utilize community rating. Under community rating the effect of a single individual becoming ill has much less impact on overall premiums because the expense is diluted and shared amongst a greater number of individuals.

THE ROLE OF THE INSURANCE COMMISSION
Even though insurance companies determine their own premium structure, they are highly regulated. Each state has a State Insurance Commission to which the companies must report at least annually. Insurance companies must also request approval for rate (premium) increases from the commission. If the commission decides the premiums are excessive, the rate increase will be denied. One of the duties of the State Insurance Commission is to protect patients from price gouging.

TYPES OF COVERAGE
Typically, there are three primary types of insurance coverage: basic, comprehensive, and catastrophic.

BASIC INSURANCE POLICIES provide fundamental requirements. They often don't cover preventive and routine care procedures. Due to their limited coverage, the premiums are generally lower than those for comprehensive policies.

COMPREHENSIVE INSURANCE POLICIES provide the most complete coverage, hence they are typically the most expensive. There are many variations on this type of policy.

CATASTROPHIC INSURANCE POLICIES (once referred to as major medical) usually involve coverage only after a large deductible is satisfied. Because the yearly deductible is so high (deductibles can be in the range of $3,000 to $5,000) the subscriber pays for routine care. The insurance companies are gambling that you will stay healthy enough that you will not exceed your deductible. This policy is ideal for the healthy individual who has enough money to cover routine care yet wants to be insured against the financial burden associated with catastrophic illnesses. These policies usually have the least expensive premiums.

Whether you have a basic, comprehensive, or catastrophic policy, you should understand your contract completely and know what is covered and what is excluded. Otherwise, you could find yourself not covered for a specific service or procedure that you need and had thought was covered under your policy. Research is your powerful tool. Coverage and exclusions differ from policy to policy and insurance company to insurance company, so you owe it to yourself to discover by how much.

Knowing your insurance coverage is vital to ensuring that you obtain the health care you need.

KNOW THE INSURANCE LANGUAGE BEFORE PLAYING THE GAME

As with any specialized business, insurance has devised its own language. In order to understand your insurance policies and to speak more efficiently and effectively with your company's representatives, you should familiarize yourself with the following terms and their definitions. Speaking and using insurance language correctly can be a powerful tool. When the insurance company believes that you are a knowledgeable consumer, they tend to show more respect when listening to your concerns and issues. The following is a list of terms with which you should be familiar.

Co-insurance—The portion of the bill that you pay. If the insurance company pays 80 percent of a bill, then you co-insure for the remaining 20 percent.

Co-payment—The fixed dollar amount that you pay directly to the caregiver at each office visit. Co-payments typically range from $5 to $25.

Covered dependent—An individual, usually a spouse or child, who receives benefits through your policy.

Deductible—The fixed dollar amount that you pay out of pocket each year before the insurance carrier begins to pay any of the charges.

Exclusions—Illnesses and treatments not covered by your insurance company. Exclusions can include routine care such as pregnancy, yearly physical exams, etc., or more complicated care such as infertility treatments.

Experimental—Procedures, treatments, equipment, other medical devices, drugs, etc., that are not currently recognized by the insurance company (not necessarily by the medical profession) as having been thoroughly tested and proven effective.

Maximum benefits—The maximum reimbursement for medical expenses per year or per lifetime that your insurance company will pay for you.

Pre-authorization—Approval obtained from the insurance company prior to performing certain procedures. An authorization number must be submitted with the bill for it to be paid.

Pre-existing condition—Medical condition, illness, or injury occurring prior to signing up for insurance.

Referral—One health care professional sending you to another health care professional for assistance.

Subscriber—The person (usually you, your spouse, or your parent) who contracts with the insurance company.

Usual, customary, reasonable—Typical fee charged by other physicians in the community for the same service.

Your understanding of these terms will help you when you are dealing with your insurance coverage.

WHAT HAPPENS WHEN YOU CHANGE INSURANCE PROGRAMS

If you have an individual policy and decide to switch insurance companies, you may have to meet the application qualifications for the new company. This means that you may have to undergo a physical exam and be subjected to a pre-existing conditions clause. Therefore, if you have developed a chronic illness or other condition since you last applied for insurance, you may have difficulty qualifying for a new individual insurance policy. It is important that if possible you always obtain the new insurance coverage before you give up your old coverage.

When an employer switches to a new group policy, it usually has no effect on the continuity of your coverage, except that the new insurance company may enforce a waiting period for coverage of pre-existing conditions. If this is the case, you may have a gap in your coverage for those conditions until the waiting period is over. The only changes you should expect to see relate to the details of the plan and how it is administered. If your employer is considering changing insurance companies, try to discuss the changes with the plan administrator before they are made.

CHANGING JOBS

Normally, your employer sponsored insurance coverage ends when you change or lose your job. There is usually a 30-day grace period during which your previous insurance coverage remains in force. If your new employer has group insurance you will become eligible for that insurance coverage. However, you will most likely have to wait until after your probationary period before you become eligible for the insurance. Then you will also have to deal with the waiting period for pre-existing conditions to minimize preexisting illness exclusions.

To ease the burden of a gap in insurance coverage, Congress, as part of the Consolidated Omnibus Budget Reconciliation Act of 1986 (COBRA), established that employers with 20 or more employees and insurance companies must allow the former employee to extend coverage for up to 18 months after the job termination. The employee must file for COBRA coverage within 30 days of losing his job and then must pay for the entire insurance premium. The purpose of COBRA is to guarantee that an employee has health care insurance during the time it takes to find a new job and qualify for another insurance policy. Continuing COBRA coverage after finding a new job is also a way for you to keep your insurance coverage for pre-existing conditions during the probationary period of your new job and during the waiting period of your new insurance coverage.

Because the COBRA protection was not considered adequate, Congress passed the Health Insurance Portability and Accountability Act (HIPA) of 1996. This law is designed to guarantee health insurance coverage for individuals who lose their coverage due to termination or change in employment. HIPA took effect in July, 1997, and applies to companies who sponsor group health plans and have two or more employees. Employers issue certificates to employees who are leaving. They can then take these certificates to a new employer to reduce the pre-existing waiting period. Insurance companies are prevented from denying coverage based on the health status of an individual and must renew policies as long as the premium is paid.

WHAT IF YOUR INSURANCE IS CANCELED?

You may have your insurance policy suddenly canceled if an insurance carrier decides to no longer cover the risk group for which you are a member. If your policy is canceled without warning or justification, it may be necessary to seek legal council to protect your rights. You should at least determine if the company will cover you for the period during which you look for other coverage.

MAKING AN INTELLIGENT CHOICE

With this background on health insurance it is time to focus on choosing the right plan for you. This requires that you be a skillful shopper. For each policy on your shopping list, there are several important issues to compare:

AFFORDABILITY Does the policy fit within your budget? Be aware that there are two types of costs to you, the obvious and the hidden. The most obvious cost is the premium. This will vary depending on the number of people to be insured, their ages, and the type of coverage you choose. The major hidden costs include the deductible, the co-pay, the co-insurance, and the life-time maximum benefit. For example, if you go to a provider for a $100 visit, with a $10 co-pay and 50 percent co-insurance, you pay $55 and your insurance company pays $45. And if you have a $500 deductible, the insurance company pays nothing until you have satisfied this deductible. As this example illustrates, hidden costs are substantial.

> ### INSIDER'S HINT
> *The lowest monthly payment is not necessarily the best or most afford-able policy.*

ALTERNATIVE MEDICINE Alternative medicine is gaining greater recognition and acceptance within the society. As a result, insurance companies now cover some alternative care expenses, such as acupuncture and chiropractic. However, other alternative forms of medicine are not routinely covered.

BENEFITS What is covered under the policy? Do the benefits meet your current health needs?

DEPENDENTS How well are dependents (children and spouse) covered under the policy? Who are considered dependents?

EMERGENCY CARE Is emergency room care covered? How far away is the covered emergency care? What if you cannot get to your company's emergency room in time? Who pays?

ELECTIVE PROCEDURES What elective procedures, if any, are covered? Are treatments such as plastic surgery, infertility, or impotence covered?

EXCLUSIONS Are there exclusions? Does the policy cover what you want it to cover including maternity, dental, vision, hearing, rehabilitation, and psychiatric care? These are not always standard elements of insurance contracts. Many companies offer additional policies at additional cost for covering these services.

EXPENSIVE TREATMENTS Policies cover ongoing or expensive procedures differently. For example, there may be yearly limits placed on physical therapy. Some extremely expensive treatments, such as organ and bone marrow transplants, may not be covered under the policy or may be severely limited. Insurance plans that do provide for this type of care often have a lifetime limit for reimbursement. If you desire coverage for this type of care, you need to carefully review the policy.

FAMILY HISTORY By knowing your family's medical history you may be better able to anticipate your future medical needs. Many diseases such as arthritis, diabetes, breast cancer, heart disease, and stroke occur at a high frequency in certain families. You may require special monitoring or treatment to prevent the onset of disease or complications. Therefore, it is important to select a policy that would provide good coverage were you to get one of your family's diseases.

GATEKEEPER SYSTEM The gatekeeper system is designed to reduce "unnecessary" care by having a single doctor decide what consultations, tests, or treatments are indicated. This system requires you to give up control over your health care choices in exchange for lower premiums.

If an insurance program uses gatekeepers, do your best to find out the following:

1. How is the gatekeeper paid?
2. If gatekeepers send patients for too many referrals or specialized tests can they be fired or do they make less money than their colleagues who order fewer referrals or tests?
3. Do gatekeepers have financial incentives for limiting usage of medical resources?
4. What can you do to get additional care if you disagree with the gatekeepers decisions? What are your rights?

5. Is there a gag rule, financial disincentive, or profiling system in effect that might limit your doctor from fully disclosing your health care options?

Accreditation lists and other information about gatekeeper-directed managed care organizations are available at 1-888-275-7585 or on the web at www.ncqa.org.

HEALTH MAINTENANCE COVERAGE Is there coverage for routine yearly physical exams, lab tests, vision and dental care, mammograms, osteoporosis bone density evaluations? Many policies offer additional payment plans for covering these aspects of care.

HMO Is the plan an HMO? Do you like the physicians in the HMO? Is your current physician in the HMO? If not, you will be required to select a new primary care doctor. Does the HMO have a hospital nearby where you can seek emergency or inpatient care?

MATERNITY Is maternity care covered? You may be surprised at the limitations placed on your policy?

MAXIMUM BENEFITS Are the maximum benefits divided into yearly or lifetime benefits? For instance, if you require physical therapy for a chronic injury, you may be covered for only $500 per year. At $80 per visit that is only six visits. Anything after that you must pay. If you have a paralyzing injury, you may be covered only up to $500,000. After that, you pay all of the costs associated with illness. This would probably bankrupt the average individual.

MENTAL HEALTH Are mental health visits covered? If yes, what is covered?

OUT-OF-TOWN COVERAGE Out-of-town care may not be covered by all policies. Because the out-of-town doctors are not usually preferred providers you might have to pay for all routine care. If you become ill when you're out of town, most policies cover emergency care without obtaining prior authorization from the insurance company. If you are uncertain, call the company and have them fax an authorization to you or the out-of-town doctor to assure yourself that the bill will be paid.

PPO Does the insurance plan use a preferred provider organization panel. "Preferred" does not mean the insurance company went out and found the best doctors and signed them up. It means the insurance carrier got the doctor to agree to a sizable discount in rates and/or that the company believes that the doctor does not order too many expensive tests. Be cautious when examining who is on the preferred provider list. Make sure there is an adequate selection of doctors to choose from. Most importantly, be sure the doctors you are currently seeing are on the preferred provider list.

If your doctor is not a preferred provider, you will have to pay the difference between his rate and what the insurance company will cover. If the insurance covers preferred providers at 80 percent and non-preferred providers at 50 percent, a $50 visit to a non-preferred provider would cost $25.

PRE-EXISTING CONDITIONS Does the policy include pre-existing conditions language? If you are accepted with a pre-existing illness, is there a waiting period before your pre-existing illness is covered? Be sure to clarify these details before you accept any policy. You may be able to get the waiting period eliminated if you are presently in good health. An insurance agent can help you submit the necessary information to try to have any limitations on a pre-existing condition waved.

PREVENTIVE CARE This is the same as health maintenance coverage.

RELIABILITY Many new insurance companies and managed care groups are forming. It is important to ensure that the company you sign up with will be around for years to come. Ask your agent about the stability and equity of the company that you are considering. You can also get this information from the state insurance commissioner.

SPECIALISTS The trend in medicine is to make it more difficult for you to see a specialist. Does the insurance company require that you first see a gatekeeper or generalist before you can be seen by a specialist?

WORK RELATED ILLNESSES AND INJURIES Most people are not aware that health insurance policies do not cover medical expenses resulting from work related accidents or diseases. Most employers carry labor and industry (L & I) insurance. This arrangement works fine as long as L & I agrees to pay the bills. But if they refuse to pay or authorize care, which is not uncommon, you are left with either paying the bill while you do battle with the L & I administrator. Some health insurance policies will pay for work related claims if they have been denied payment by L & I. If you are willing to pay a higher premium, most insurance plans will offer coverage that even includes work related illnesses.

Once you become a knowledgeable consumer, understand some of the less publicized or hidden issues in insurance shopping, and have created a shopping list, you can work with your insurance agent or company to select the policy that best meets your needs and fits within your budget. Exercise 16-1 will help you with this task.

Selecting Health Insurance

The questions in this exercise will help you to compare health insurance plans. For each category, write in the information for the health insurance plan you are considering under the "Your Plan" category. You can obtain this information by contacting the insurance company, reading a benefits book, or asking your insurance agent.

Evaluate each item by assigning a plus sign (+) if the plan meets your needs for that particular item or a minus sign (-) if it does not meet your needs. When you have finished, go back through the list and identify the five elements that you consider to be most important. For example, a person might consider premium amount, preventive services, vision benefits, self referral options, and location to be of primary importance. Look to see if you put a plus or minus next to the elements that you deem to be most important. If you put all pluses, the plan most likely meets your needs. However, if you put all minuses, the plan is not right for you. If you have a mixture of pluses and minuses, you will need to carefully consider the plan in comparison with others before selecting it.

Make photocopies of this exercise if you are looking at more than one plan.

	Your Plan	Meets Needs? (+ or−)

TYPE OF PLAN

1. Is the plan fee-for-service or capitated (prepaid) managed care?

2. Is the policy a group or individual policy?

COST OF PLAN (AFFORDABILITY)

1. How much is the monthly premium?

2. How much is the yearly deductible?

3. If there are co-payments for visits, how much are they?

4. If there are co-payments for prescriptions, how much are they?

5. If there is co-insurance, how much is it?

6. What is the lifetime maximum benefit amount?

7. If there is an out-of-pocket maximum amount, how much is it?

EXERCISE 16-1

Selecting Health Insurance *(cont.)*

	Your Plan	Meets Needs? (+ or–)

PREEXISTING CONDITIONS (PRIOR ILLNESSES)

1. Is there a preexisting conditions clause?

2. If there is a waiting period for preexisting conditions, how long is it?

3. Must you submit to a health physical before coverage is approved?

DEPENDENTS

1. Who qualifies as dependents?

PLAN COVERAGE (BENEFITS)

1. Are routine physical exams for adults covered?

2. Are screening exams—pap smears, mammograms, and prostate exams—covered?

3. Are maternity benefits covered?

4. Is well-baby care covered?

5. Are inpatient physician surgical services covered?

6. Are outpatient physician surgical services covered?

7. Is an anesthetist covered?

8. Is a second surgical opinion covered?

9. Are inpatient physician visits covered?

10. Are outpatient physician visits covered?

11. Are inpatient diagnostic x-ray and laboratory services covered?

12. Are outpatient diagnostic x-ray and laboratory services covered?

13. Are physical, occupational, and speech therapists covered?

14. Is spinal manipulation covered?

15. Is hospital room and board covered?

EXERCISE 16-1

Selecting Health Insurance *(cont.)*

	Your Plan	Meets Needs? (+ or−)
17. Are emergency room visits covered? Is a co-pay required?		
18. Are ambulance services covered?		
19. Is durable medical and surgical equipment covered?		
20. Are artificial limbs, eyes, and other prostheses covered?		
21. Are hearing exams covered?		
22. Are hearing aids covered? If yes, how many?		
23. Are annual vision exams covered?		
24. Are contact lenses, glass lenses, and frames covered? If yes, how much?		
25. Are mental health benefits available? How many visits are allowed per year?		
26. Are substance abuse programs covered? Inpatient? Outpatient?		
27. Are alternative care providers covered?		
28. Is home health care covered? If yes, for how long?		
29. Is hospice care covered?		
30. Are skilled nursing facilities covered? Is there a maximum number of days available per year?		
31. Is cosmetic surgery covered? Medically necessary vs. elective?		
32. Is reconstructive breast surgery covered?		
33. Are temporomandibular joint disorders (TMJ) covered?		
34. Are human organ transplants covered? Is there a lifetime maximum dollar amount for transplants?		
35. Are prescription drugs covered? If yes, is there a co-payment amount?		
36. Are mail ordered drug services covered?		
37. How is out-of-town care covered?		
38. Do you have worker's compensation? If no, can you purchase a policy rider?		

Selecting Health Insurance *(cont.)*

	Your Plan	Meets Needs? (+ or–)

PHYSICIAN CHOICE

1. Can you see the physician you desire?

2. Must you choose from a panel of physicians?

3. Must you select a primary care giver from whom you seek most services?

4. Does your PCP act as a gatekeeper? Who coordinates your care?

5. How often can you change your PCP in a year?

6. Can you self refer for routine visits, such as Pap smears or vision exams?

7. Can you self refer to specialists? If yes, will it cost you more?

8. How are the physicians reimbursed under the plan?

CONVENIENCE

1. Are the plan's physicians' offices conveniently located near your home or work?

2. Are the plan's hospitals conveniently located near your home or work?

PLAN ADMINISTRATION (BUSINESS DETAILS)

1. Is the insurance benefits booklet easy to read and understand?

2. Does the booklet disclose all of the insurance's limitations and exclusions?

3. Do you have to file a claim with the plan or does the doctor do that for you? If no, is it easy to file a claim with the plan?

4. Does the plan have an acceptable grievance process if you have a problem?

5. Does the plan coordinate benefits with other plans for you?

6. Is it easy for the plan to cancel your coverage? How many days notice must they give you?

7. Is your health plan local or will you be dealing with someone in another part of the country?

Chapter 17

The Medical Bill

One day in early june, Julie Waters received a bill from a collection agency for $1,240 (plus interest!) for doctor bills incurred over the previous nine months. Julie was terribly confused by the bill and believed it must be a mistake. Julie had insurance coverage and assumed that the insurance company was always timely in its payments to her doctor. Her doctor's staff had never indicated to her that they weren't receiving payment.

The same day Julie received the bill, she telephoned her doctor's office. No, the collection agency bill was no mistake, they said. Julie's insurance company had not paid any bills since October. The doctor's staff had billed the insurance company several times and been denied payment every time. The doctor's staff told Julie they had no recourse but to send her account to collection.

Julie immediately called her insurance company and explained her problem to the customer service representative. The rep asked for Julie's member number and confirmed that no claims had been paid on her behalf. She asked Julie if there had been any changes in her employment status since the problem began. "Why yes, I retired October first." "Oh, that might explain it," the rep said. "You do realize that at retirement you were given a new member number that identifies you as a retiree. Perhaps your doctor's office is still submitting claims to us by using your old member number."

Sure enough, Julie called and found out the doctor's staff was still using her old number instead of the new one. She asked the staff to resubmit all the claims using her new member number. Julie was rightfully upset that this had happened to her. She had been a patient of this doctor for the last 20 years. Before she hung-up, she couldn't help but say, "Why did you have to let my account go to a collection agency? I'm a long-time patient with no history of non-payment. Didn't it ever occur to you to just pick up the phone and call me or the insurance company to find out what the problem was?"

MAKING SENSE OF THE BILL

The bill, or statement of your account, is a notice that you receive either from the physician or your insurance company telling you how much is owed by you or your insurance company for services performed. Your doctor or insurance company may use different terminology, but common items found on a medical bill include:

- Personal information
- Closing date (date the bill was generated)
- Payment date (date the bill must be paid)
- Amount due (account balance)
- Percent of finance charges (interest payable on overdue amount)
- Date of service
- Doctor
- Description of service
- Place of service
- Diagnostic code (billing number that precisely describes service rendered)
- Charges
- Insurance payment amount (amount the insurance company will pay)
- Disallowed amount (amount the insurance company will not pay)
- Due from patient (amount the patient must pay the doctor)

BILLING PRACTICES

For an office visit, you will most likely receive a single bill. The bill will be itemized, and any individual charges, such as lab tests and procedures, supplies used, and physician's time, will be listed separately. For outpatient procedures, you may get two separate bills. One bill will be for the technical component or the facility's fee and the other bill will be for the professional component or doctor's time. For example, when you have a chest x-ray you may be billed by the x-ray facility for the technician taking and processing the x-ray film, and then billed by the physician for interpreting the x-ray.

DOES YOUR DOCTOR KNOW HOW MUCH SHE CHARGES?

Probably not. She may have a general idea of the charges, but most likely she cannot tell you how much your visit will cost. The book-keeper should be able to provide the approximate range of charges for the doctor's services. Your specific charges may then depend on modifications related to your particular insurance program.

Doctors negotiate their contracts with the different insurance companies, so a doctor can have different charge schedules for each insurance company. Therefore, the doctor can perform the same service for two different patients and bill the patients completely different charges depending on their insurance coverage. A list of your negotiated insurance charges can also be obtained from the book-keeper. To avoid sticker shock, you may want to ask for a list of typical charges prior to your office visit. This allows you time to call other offices and compare prices if your insurance company doesn't require you to see a particular physician.

WHO GETS BILLED AND WHEN?

The contracts doctors have with the different insurance companies, Medicare, Medicaid, and Labor and Industry often require the doctors to bill the insurance provider directly, unless the charges are:
- not covered by the insurance,
- part of the deductible, or
- a co-payment to be paid by the patient.

Even though the physician may bill your insurance directly, the doctor might send you a bill to inform you what has been submitted for payment by your insurance. This bill should indicate somewhere on it that it is for your records only and no payment is required at this time. Typically, your insurance company will also send you an explanation of benefits statement. This statement indicates the service billed for by your doctor, the service charge, and the dollar amount your insurance company has paid out on your behalf.

If your doctor doesn't bill your insurance company, but instead bills you, most likely you will receive the bill within 30 days after the visit. It is very rare that you would be handed a bill as you leave the office after a visit. Most offices send bills on a regular schedule and to allow time to collect and process all necessary information. If you expect a bill within 30 days but do not get one, it would be appropriate to call the physician's billing office to inquire about it. However, under the law, doctors are not required to bill within 30 days and may actually take as long as they like to bill you.

Sometimes you will never receive a bill at all. Many HMOs and other managed care plans that operate under a monthly capitated fee do not bill patients. The reason for this is due to the nature of the HMO. Because you as an enrollee are paying on a monthly basis, you are guaranteed care for covered services under the HMO contract. Therefore, it would be a waste of time and money for the HMO to "bill" you for services you have already paid for through your monthly fee.

WHEN SHOULD YOU PAY?

If your doctor bills the insurance company directly you will not need to pay anything if the company covers all charges. However, if you are responsible for total or partial payment, your payment is usually due within 30 days of receipt of your account statement from the doctor. Sometimes, but very rarely, you may be asked to pay at the time of the visit. To best understand when you need to pay an account, ask your doctor's billing staff.

WHAT CAN GO WRONG?

Any number of problems can occur when you are dealing with complicated computer programs, insurance contracts, and humans who can make mistakes. Some of the most common billing problems are:

INCORRECT CHARGES The doctor's office might make a mistake in the amount that they charge for a procedure or even charge you for the wrong procedure.

INCORRECT POSTINGS A billing clerk might accidentally post charges or payments to your account that are not yours or even post charges or payments that are yours to another person's account.

DUPLICATE BILLS FOR THE SAME SERVICE Because most offices have automatic billing systems, a late payment may not arrive in time to prevent the system from generating the duplicate bill. If you believe your bill is already paid, just call the billing staff to confirm that your payment was received and properly posted to your account. Also, there could have been a posting error, which resulted in you getting a second bill.

INSURANCE REIMBURSEMENT PROBLEMS The problem might lie with your insurance company and not the doctor's billing staff. It could be that your insurance company is slow to process claims and pay benefits. If your doctor needs to collect on his accounts to pay salaries and bills, he might bill you directly and then have you deal with your insurance company. If you encounter this situation, then you may have to pay the doctor's bill and pursue your insurance company for reimbursement.

In any of these instances, the best way to handle the problem is to call your doctor's billing staff. Explain the situation to them in a concise and polite manner. Through patience and diligence you and the billing staff should be able to come to a resolution. If your account is complicated by multiple visits, multiple bills, and even multiple insurances, it is often best to just allow extra time at your visit to sit down and review your account with the billing staff.

RESOLVING GRIEVANCES

If you do not agree with your bill, there are several steps that you can pursue.

- Review the back of your bill. It should provide detailed information on how to dispute charges. It should also state how long you have to bring grievances to the attention of the doctor, insurance company, or outside mediator.
- Contact the doctor's billing staff and go over the bill together. Perhaps there was a mistake or error.
- Contact the doctor or clinic manager if you and the billing staff cannot come to an agreement concerning your bill. The physician or clinic manager will then decide if the bill was appropriate or if any changes need to be made to the bill.
- Call the subscriber support number at your insurance carrier and discuss your bill with a claims administrator. The claims administrator will be able to mediate on your behalf with the doctor's staff or clinic manager if you do not agree with the bill amount.
- Review the grievance procedures outlined in your insurance contract. These will tell you how to resolve a dispute with

your insurance company and the timetable in which it must be completed.

- Contact the grievance department of the local medical society, as a last resort. You can present your case to them and they will try to mediate a solution with the physician or clinic manager.

When you are disputing a bill or claim, there are procedures you should adhere to protect yourself during the process.

- Detail your dispute in a letter and mail it to your doctor or insurance company. Writing it down protects your rights and requires the doctor or insurance company to address the problem.
- Write down the facts, as you see them, in a log or diary during the entire grievance process. Refer to the log when you are discussing your problems with the different people, so that you can present a concise picture of the dispute.
- Write down the date, time, name of individual contacted, and information discussed during office and telephone conversations with the billing staff, the doctor, or insurance company.
- Keep copies of your bills, explanation of benefits' statements, checks, bank statements, and all correspondence between you and the doctor or insurance company.

If the situation escalates to a legal matter, you will have all of the necessary information. Exercise 17-1 will help you to get organized.

DEALING WITH A COLLECTION AGENCY?

A physician has the right to proceed with legal means to collect his bill. Your account may be sent to a collection agency if you have chosen to not pay a disputed bill. From then on, you must deal with the collection agency and can no longer pay your bill directly to the doctor's office. If you have been turned over to a collection agency, call your local credit assistance bureau or attorney for advice.

The Fair Debt Collection Practices Act of 1978 covers the practices of third-party debt collectors and attorneys who regularly collect debts for others. The physician (credit grantor) may be answerable for the acts and practices of the collection agency (debt collector) depending on the circumstances and, in some cases, on state laws. Generally the collection agency may communicate with the patient (debtor) between 8 A.M. and 9 P.M. local time of the patient. The collection agency may communicate with the patient at work, except when the collection agency knows or has reason to know that the employer prohibits such communication. If the patient notifies the collection agency in writing that he refuses to pay and wants communication to stop, the collection agency must stop communicating with the patient, except to advise the patient of possible actions:

1. the collection efforts will be terminated, or
2. the collection agency may undertake specified remedies that are ordinarily invoked by the collector, such as filing a lawsuit.

IF YOU DON'T GET BETTER DO YOU STILL HAVE TO PAY?

Satisfaction in the arena of medical care is difficult to define. There are many reasons for not getting better. You may have a different definition of satisfactory care than your physician. You may believe that satisfaction comes by having the disease totally eradicated, but your doctor might be satisfied with just slowing the progression of the disease and treating it as a chronic condition that requires routine health maintenance. Therefore, satisfaction guaranteed is not a concept that is usually applied when it comes to paying a doctor's bill. Unless the physician made a contract with you that if you did not improve you would not have to pay, then you still need to pay your bill. Is this fair? Perhaps not. But it is the way the system currently works.

Resolving a Billing Dispute

Keeping copies of bills, insurance statements, canceled checks, and all correspondence, as well as documenting telephone or office conversations, will be of great help if a billing dispute occurs. If it progresses to a legal matter, you will need all of this information and documentation.

FACTS ABOUT THE BILL

Date Service Provided_____

Physician Who Provided Service_____

Place Where Service Provided_____

Type of Service Provided_____

Date Bill Issued_____

Date Bill Due_____

Total Amount Due_____

Amount Paid, if any_____

Balance Due_____

BILL DISPUTE

State briefly why you disagree with this particular bill_____

_____

_____

_____

_____

_____

EXERCISE 17-1

Resolving a Billing Dispute *(cont.)*

RESOLUTION PROCESS

To discuss a billing dispute, you might initially contact any of the following individuals: physician's bookkeeper, health care provider, or insurance company. As a last resort, you may wish to contact the medical society grievance committee, credit assistance bureau, or an attorney.

Name and Position of Individual _____

Contact By Telephone, Letter or In Person_____

Date & Time of Contact_____

Briefly summarize your conversation or attach letter_____

_____

_____

_____

_____

_____

_____

_____

If contact was by letter, when and what was the response (attach letter)

_____

_____

_____

_____

Any other comments or notes _____

_____

_____

_____

_____

Chapter 18

Your Medical Record

Elaine Smith moved away from her hometown 10 years ago. When she arrived in her new city she found a new physician. At the first visit he recommended that she have her medical records transferred. However, she was very busy unpacking, starting a new job, and caring for her family so she neglected to have her medical records transferred. She rationalized that she had always been in good health and therefore thought the records wouldn't contain any particular vital information. The only medical care that she had ever required had been at the time of her children's birth, including an elective hysterectomy after her fourth child.

One evening after returning from the movies with her family, Elaine began experiencing sharp pains in her right lower abdomen. This increased so severely over the next two hours that her husband took her to the local emergency room. Elaine was asked if she had her appendix removed at the time of her hysterectomy. She couldn't remember. That night both the emergency room staff and her husband frantically attempted to obtain her old medical records. Unfortunately, the hospital that performed her surgery had closed down; the records were on microfiche and could not be rapidly obtained. Also, her previous physician had long since retired. That night Elaine's pain steadily increased. Her white blood cell count was normal but her fever persisted. A preliminary diagnosis of appendicitis was rendered and surgery was performed. At the time of surgery, the doctors discovered that Elaine's appendix had been removed so they just closed her up.

Forty-eight hours later Elaine's abdominal pain and fever resolved. The doctors concluded that Elaine had suffered from a gastrointestinal virus or food poisoning which mimicked appendicitis (not an uncommon occurrence). The next week, Elaine's medical records arrived having been retrieved from microfiche. Sure enough, they confirmed that her appendix had been removed electively during the hysterectomy. Elaine endured a surgery, an uncomfortable recovery period, and two weeks of lost wages—all of which could have been avoided if she had known her past medical history and had obtained a copy of past medical records.

THE ROLE OF MEDICAL RECORDS

Your medical record provides a description of each encounter with your health care provider. The records contain your medical history, the provider's notes regarding your symptoms and complaints, examination findings, test results, consultation reports, treatment plans, and any other piece of information your provider determines is appropriate to document.

Every time you visit a physician, hospital, or therapist, the activity is documented in a medical record. That means you have a medical record at every doctor's office you have visited. Additionally, every hospital at which you have been treated or admitted for both inpatient and outpatient services maintains medical records.

There are three primary reasons for maintaining medical records. First, it is a record that allows your doctor to review previous problems and treatments and use that information to monitor your progress and alter the treatment plan as indicated. Second, the record is a historical document that communicates your medical information to others. It is especially useful when you see a physician for the first time. Third, it is a medical-legal document that records the decision-making process and what was discussed with the patient in the event of a malpractice lawsuit, disability settlement, or other legal action.

WHO OWNS YOUR MEDICAL RECORD?

This is often a confusing issue. The health care provider owns the medical records. Even though you or your insurance company pay for the office visits and treatments, the provider (your doctor, for instance) creates the record and, as granted under state and federal licensing regulations, owns the records.

REVIEWING OR COPYING YOUR MEDICAL RECORDS

Even though you do not own your record, you have the right to examine and obtain a copy of it. When you request a copy of your record, the doctor has up to 15 days to provide you with the records. If there is a delay beyond this, the provider must notify you of the delay. The provider may charge a "reasonable" fee that is defined and modified by your state health care authority. In Washington State, for example, this was defined in 1996 as a $16 flat fee for clerical searching and handling, $.69 per page for the first 30 pages of records, and a $.53 per page after the 30th page. The provider does not have to give you the copy of your record until the fee for copying or certification of the record has been paid.

A provider may deny you access to your own health care information if:

- It may be injurious to you (in the opinion of the provider).
- It may violate other confidences, such as another person's psychiatric information, HIV status, etc.
- It could endanger the life or safety of any individual.
- The record is compiled solely for administrative, litigation, or quality assurance purposes
- Access is prohibited by the law.

If upon reviewing your record you find what you consider to be a mistake, do you have the right to request a change in the record? Generally, the answer is yes. If you request a change in your record, a health care provider should make the correction if it indeed is an error. If the provider refuses to make the correction, then you have the right to insert into your record a statement of disagreement with the information.

IS YOUR PRIVACY BEING PROTECTED?

States have enacted laws that protect your privacy and your rights regarding medical records. Generally, these laws state that health care providers must not disclose health information to any person without a written patient authorization. Also, the provider must document each disclosure, *except to third party payers*. This is a very important aspect of your health insurance contract. It will very likely state that the insurance company can obtain your records to document that the services billed for were indeed performed. This clause serves as a blanket release form for the insurance company to obtain the records that they feel they need to review in order to validate the claim.

There are a few circumstances in which a provider may release information without your written authorization. These include:

- To another health care provider who is treating you and needs information to help with your care.
- To another person for health education, planning, quality assurance, peer review, actuarial, legal, financial, or administrative purpose where your confidentiality is maintained.
- To minimize an imminent danger to you, the patient.
- For bona fide research purposes where your identity is not revealed.
- To auditors or to legal authorities if you are in jail.

Others may also have access to your medical records. Professional and nonprofessional medical staff in hospitals or clinics will have access to your records. Additionally, quality assurance committees, joint commission inspection teams, and state licensure reviewers will have access to medical records in hospitals. A health care provider must also disclose patient health information to public health authorities or law enforcement agencies when required by law, or to a court or attorneys when required by a compulsory legal process. However, disclosure to family members and to previous health care providers cannot be made without patient consent. Also, release of information to your employer or creditors can only be done with your written consent. As you can see, you do not have total privacy in regards to your medical records.

HOW DO YOU PROTECT YOURSELF?

In order for a physician to accurately diagnose and treat you, you must give complete and honest information, even if it is embarrassing. If you discuss something that you do not want in your record, request that no entry be made of the discussion. For example, you go to your family physician for a routine exam, and end up disclosing that in college you routinely used illegal drugs. This is information that you definitely do not want your boss, spouse, or even the insurance company to know about. However, it is crucial information to your doctor because it may affect your health. Your options would be to just pay for the office visit and not have your insurance company billed for this visit or you can ask that the record of your illegal drug use be kept separate from the rest of your chart. Another option is to have it labeled in your chart as something that should never be released without first talking to you.

For the most part, however, you do not need to ask your doctor to keep two sets of records for you. To release your medical records, except in the cases above, the provider needs to obtain written authorization from you. This release form must:

- be in writing—dated and signed by the patient or by the legal guardian, if the patient is a minor or legally incompetent
- identify the nature of the information to be disclosed— including the name, address, and institutional affiliation of the person to whom the information is to be disclosed
- identify the provider who is to make the disclosure

Release of information forms must contain a statement relating to the release of any part of the record that contains information pertaining to a history of mental illness or sexually transmitted disease or condition. This statement is intended to make you very aware that this type of information may be in your records and may be released.

You can obtain a release of information form from your doctor. Authorizations must be kept by the provider as part of the medical record and it must be charted that the information was disclosed to a third party. An authorization form is valid for 90 days after it is signed. After that, a new release form must be obtained from the patient.

You may revoke a written authorization at any time. However, the provider is protected if the information has already been released under a proper authorization. If the provider is still in the process of complying with the original release, you must submit the revocation in writing and ask him to stop the release of information at that time. The provider should halt the release process, but may want to notify the person requesting the information that the release is no longer valid and the records will not be forthcoming.

HOW LONG MUST MEDICAL RECORDS BE MAINTAINED?

Written medical records produced by your physician or by the hospital must be maintained 10 years from the last visit and 5 years from the date of death. Birth records must be kept for 20 years. Laboratory records and radiology imaging studies (x-rays, MRI, etc.) must be kept for 2½ years. After the mandatory period has expired then records may be destroyed. In radiology departments it is not uncommon to purge x-rays regularly. This occurs without your knowledge and without your approval. Thus, the only copy of your x-rays or imaging studies can be destroyed. For this reason, you might consider making a copy of any vital records or films. The problem with keeping your own films and records is that they can be lost or damaged easily. Therefore, an alternative solution is to have written notice placed in your medical records or x-ray films that you wish to be contacted and obtain your records or films before they are destroyed. This may be a logistical nightmare for the doctor's office or for the hospital, but it is your right.

SHOULD YOU MAINTAIN YOUR OWN PRIVATE MEDICAL RECORDS?

The answer is a most definite yes. As you learned in Chapter 8, there are several reasons for keeping your own medical records. First, it allows you to take an active role in your health care. It provides you with a means to record your own notes and interpretation of your care. Second, your records might get destroyed or inadvertently altered at your doctor's office. After all, medical records are still mostly paper, and paper burns. And even though more and more providers are using computerized records, computers crash, disks are lost, and information can be added, deleted, or changed. Third, maintaining your own records will make it much easier and efficient to establish yourself with a new physician, particularly if you are moving out of town or if some of your records are old. Finally, if you do want to get that second opinion without your primary care doctor knowing, you will be able to provide the new physician with all of the important background information without having to sign a release from your current physician.

BEGINNING YOUR OWN MEDICAL RECORD

Keeping your own medical records can prove extremely valuable if you have ever had a serious illness. Even if you have never been ill, keeping old records and x-rays may improve your care, save you from worry ,or even help you avoid an unnecessary surgery. In our opening story, Elaine Smith would have escaped a needless surgery if only she had kept her own medical records or known that she had already undergone an appendectomy. If you are extremely thorough you may desire to maintain a complete record which will include all of the items listed in Exercise 18-1 on page 281. However, most of us are not quite so organized. As a minimum, we recommend that you record the information discussed below:

HEALTH HISTORY The first step would be to complete the health history questionnaires included in this book, particularly those in Chapter 8. Make two copies of them; one that you can take to your new physician and the other to keep in your personal record.

SUMMARY OF PHYSICIAN VISITS AND HOSPITALIZATIONS Every time you visit a doctor or you are hospitalized you will want to record and summarize the visit in your personal record. This need not be complicated, particularly since most of us see a health care provider only a few times a year. However, the more you see providers the more important the record becomes. Simply record the date of the visit, who you saw, why, and what was done and discussed. This may require you to write down some information, such as blood pressure or temperature, at the time of visit. However, for the most part, just make a mental note and then record your comments and observations after the visit.

RECORD YOUR TELEPHONE CALLS. You should also document your telephone conversations with your doctor. This should be done in the same manner as for an office visit. For example, if you call after hours because of symptoms of a bladder infection and are prescribed an antibiotic over the phone, note this encounter in your record.

MEDICATIONS Keep a list of all prescribed medications and why they were prescribed. You should write down the specifics of the prescription: who prescribed the medicine, how much was prescribed, how often you are to take it, and which pharmacy issued the drug. Additionally, record any adverse reactions or side effects that you have to the medications. Also, note whether or not you felt the medication worked.

INSURANCE RECORDS AND BILLS You should also maintain copies of all bills, payments receipts, insurance statements and any other correspondence.

COPIES OF YOUR TEST RESULTS AND IMPORTANT OFFICIAL RECORDS Finally, try to obtain copies of your lab and other test results, admitting history, and physical and discharge summaries for any hospitalizations. If possible you may want to keep copies of any vital x-ray or imaging films at home. If you do this on an ongoing basis, it will not be a burden to your physician's office, with only a few pages to be copied at a time, and most likely you will not be charged.

Once you have obtained the information and started your record, keep it in a safe place. If you are maintaining a paper record, consider storing it in a fireproof safety box. If you are keeping your record on computer, consider making a backup disk to be stored in a fireproof safety box or away from your home. No matter what, the important thing is to at least keep your medical record handy, so that it is not a hassle to update it with every health care encounter.

Medical Records Checklist

The documents identified here should be included in your personal medical records.

Document	Date Included in Record (optional)
❏ Medical History Form	_____
❏ Medication Information Form	_____
❏ Symptoms Log	_____
❏ Office Visit and Telephone Log	_____
❏ Test Work-up Log	_____
❏ Copies of your records maintained by your doctor	_____
❏ Lab Results	_____
❏ Test Results	_____
❏ X-rays	_____
❏ Treatment Plans	_____
❏ Consultation Reports	_____
❏ Insurance Documents	_____
❏ Insurance Statements	_____
❏ Referrals	_____
❏ Bills	_____
❏ Canceled Checks	_____
❏ Other Relevant Correspondence	_____

Chapter 19

Medicine, Law, and Ethics

An Overview

Last year, Sam Jones was diagnosed with widely metastatic prostate cancer. Not long after, the 76 year old began to experience steadily worsening pain throughout his spine. With the cancer spreading, his doctor advised him that the cancer could not be stopped. Only morphine pills could relieve the pain.

Given the prognosis, Sam reflected on his life and his children, grandchildren, and wife. As his pain grew steadily worse, he began to worry more and more about how he would die. Sam was losing control of his life. The next time Sam saw his doctor he asked if he could get an intravenous injection of a medicine that would just end his suffering. The doctor declined and asked Sam to keep fighting. Instead of the usual 30 morphine pills for Sam, however, the doctor prescribed 100 pills, telling him that he just wanted to make sure Sam had enough to last until the next appointment. What the doctor didn't know was that Sam had begun hoarding his morphine pills during the previous three months. Consequently, Sam had about 100 extra pills at home. Two days after his doctor visit, Sam's wife found him dead in bed. Everyone assumed it had been a heart attack, and they were thankful that he didn't have to suffer any more pain.

It would have been illegal for the doctor to administer a lethal dose of medicine. In fact, it would have been considered *euthanasia*—the active ending of a life. Still, perhaps Sam's physician assisted Sam's end-of-suffering request by prescribing 70 extra morphine pills.

Then again, maybe Sam just decided on his own to stop his suffering by taking an overdose of the pills he had secretly saved up.

THE SCOPE OF THE PROBLEM

End of life decisions represent just one of the many complex ethical and legal issues that surround modern medical care. Specific laws vary greatly from state to state, so most of the information in this chapter should not be regarded as incontrovertible fact but rather as guidelines. Nevertheless, legal and ethical concerns do impact medical care, so it's important to be knowledgeable about issues you or a family member may face. If you have specific questions about the laws in your state, contact your attorney or local hospital administrator for the policies and laws that apply to your jurisdiction.

Until the 20th century, medical practice primarily involved observing disease and making the patient comfortable. Over the past 50 years, though, advances in medical technology have created new ethical, moral, economic, and public policy dilemmas. The following is a brief discussion of some of the major areas of debate.

ORGAN TRANSPLANTS Organ transplants require allocation of scant resources to those who would seem to benefit the most from the transplant. Someone has to make a decision about who can and cannot receive the benefit. This is a difficult decision at best, because those who are denied transplants face an almost certain early death.

When kidney transplantation first became available, it was viewed as an extraordinary life-saving procedure that was very expensive and involved very limited resources. As a public health policy, all patients who went onto dialysis or had a transplant were automatically eligible for Medicare. Nowadays, renal transplantation is more common and is included in most private health insurance plans.

With the advances in science and technology, doctors can now perform bone marrow transplants to save the lives of patients with many different types of cancer. Who should pay for this type of transplantation, private insurance or Medicare/Medicaid? Soon technology will allow gene transplantation for many conditions. Who should pay for this? And which conditions should be treated first? If everyone who could benefit from new treatments were covered by Medicare/ Medicaid, it could theoretically "bankrupt" the health care system.

Another issue concerning organ transplants is the availability of organs. There are currently not enough available organs to meet the needs of everyone on the transplant waiting lists. Once an organ does become available, health care professionals then have to evaluate who should get the organ. Should the transplant criteria be based on the length of time you have been waiting for an organ or the severity of your condition? One idea is to give priority to individuals who are listed as organ donors on their driver's license. Perhaps this would encourage more people to sign-up as organ donors and in turn increase the supply of organs available for transplant.

DISCONNECTION/REMOVAL OF LIFE-SUSTAINING MEDICAL DEVICES Terminating or withholding life-sustaining treatments from those seriously and chronically ill forces us to ask questions about the value and quality of life. For example, can a person who is a complete quadriplegic lead a rewarding and valuable life? (Just look at Christopher Reeves, who has become an inspiration while making great contributions to society.) Can that person still contribute to society or will he be a drain on society as he uses scarce resources to maintain his physical life. Does the patient or surrogate decision maker have the right to pull the plug on the patient's breathing apparatus even if the person is not brain dead? If yes, how should that decision be made and carried out?

GENETIC ISSUES As we gain new understanding about diseases at their most basic genetic levels, we must face the specter of discrimination against individuals who possess defective or suspect genes. Will individuals be denied jobs, health or life insurance, or other services and resources because of their genetic makeup?

REPRODUCTION ISSUES In-vitro fertilization and other embryo transfer techniques raise issues of biological versus nurturing parenthood, and in rare cases, produce "ownership" questions of frozen embryos.

EXPERIMENTAL DRUGS OR PROCEDURES Experimental treatments may offer desperate patients hope at the cost of great risk to the patient because the exact complications and side-effects are not usually known. Also, the success rate is often in doubt with experimental treatments, thus leaving us to question at what cost should we pursue these treatments.

The list of potential issues is almost endless. Interpretation of these issues is quite complex and very dependent upon personal values and ethics. As a complete and full discussion is beyond the scope of this book, we encourage you to explore these issues further on your own.

Your Rights as a Patient

Self-determination is the right to choose your own path. Unfortunately, the right of self-determination is not guaranteed by the U.S. Constitution. Otherwise, in health care situations, only you would have the right to grant or withhold consent for your medical care. Instead, there are several forces at work that may influence the care you receive.

The government, through the Food and Drug Administration, restricts access to treatments that are dangerous (thalidomide for pregnant women), unproved (the solvent DMSO), or politically charged (marijuana for medical purposes and RU483 for abortions).

Insurance companies restrict access by limiting coverage. Most alternative therapies are not covered by medical insurance policies. This is a de facto restriction because the reality is that most people cannot afford to pay for all the alternative therapy they desire out of their pockets. Even prescription drug formularies, the lists of medications for which the insurance company will pay, are limited. This intrudes on your right to determine your type of care. It is important that you review your insurance policy and know what is and is not covered. If there are deficiencies in the policy that you feel could infringe upon you health care rights, and if you cannot simply change insurance plans, lobby the insurance company and the state insurance commissioner in order to address the issues.

Informed Consent

The physician has the "duty to warn" patients of the risks, benefits, and alternatives to all of the therapies the physician prescribes. This information is usually conveyed verbally to the patient. However, when the treatment involves significant risk or a major procedure or an experimental procedure, written informed consent is required.

Informed consent involves signing a document that is written in a language the patient understands and includes the following four components:
- a description of the proposed treatment
- the expected result
- possible alternative treatments
- recognized possible serious side-effects to both the proposed and alternative treatments, which incorporates no treatment as an option.

When admitted to a hospital, patients usually sign a consent for general hospital care in addition to a consent for the specific procedure they will receive. If an emergency, when the patient cannot understand or grant informed consent and no surrogate is available to make health care decisions, consent can be waived and care administered in order to ensure the patient's wellness.

YOUR RIGHT TO COMPETENT CARE

In almost all medical situations, the doctor and patient must choose between several options: which tests to perform, medicines to use, procedures to do, or whether to just wait and see what happens. If the end result is a cure or improved health, we seldom question whether the decisions that were made were the best. However, if the results are poor, it is human nature to question the doctor's decisions. It is difficult to accept that bad things happen to good people who are well cared for.

Despite all of the advances in medicine and science, people become ill and die through no fault of their own or their doctor. For example, a difficult childbirth may result in fetal brain damage (lack of oxygen to the newborn's brain) and then cerebral palsy. This can occur even when every possible precaution and the best medical care is delivered to the mother and newborn.

MISTAKES

Mistakes are a reality of medicine and occur daily. They have always existed and will continue to exist so long as medicine is practiced by "imperfect" human beings. While mistakes sometimes lead to new insights and breakthroughs, many of these mistakes sadly result in harm to the patient.

Realizing that most mistakes are not the result of negligence or incompetence, the question comes down to: When is it justified to consider that a bad outcome is the result of incompetence or negligence and perhaps take legal action?

Bad outcomes that do involve errors can be classified as:
- Oversights or Honest Mistakes
- Compounded Errors
- Incompetence or Negligence

OVERSIGHTS unfortunately occur more frequently than expected. Fortunately, most are discovered before the patient is irreparably harmed. These honest mistakes usually occur because of one of the following:
- Incorrect assumptions
- Lack of information or knowledge, particularly of the patient's past medical history
- Incorrect judgments
- Poor focus due to being tired or ill, etc.
- System errors

The following **honest mistake** is an example of an oversight made by good doctors. An x-ray of the abdomen is performed to examine the bowel and stomach because of indigestion. In the corner of the film a small lung tumor is present but not seen by the radiologist or the primary care doctor. The doctors are focused on the abdomen, looking for a problem there, and thus have "tunnel vision." A year later the patient develops a cough. This time a chest x-ray is performed and the cancer is found. The doctor looks back at the old films and only then realizes that the cancer had been present a year earlier.

COMPOUNDED ERRORS Sometimes bad results can be caused by compounded errors. One such example occurred in a 74-year-old woman with digestive problems secondary to her diabetes. Her primary care physician (PCP) refers her to a gastroenterologist who places her on a medication to improve the slow motility in her intestine. The woman then returns to the care of her primary care physician. She develops a rare side effect of the medication, an involuntary movement of her head and tongue. However, her family physician does not recognize it as a complication of her medications. Instead, he attributes the movements disorder to neurological problems related to the diabetes. Unfortunately, the gastroenterologist who was aware that this medication can cause this type of complication was not contacted by the family physician. The gastroenterologist had never warned the patient of this complication because it is rare. In addition, the gastroenterologist and the patient never saw each other again because the intestinal problem had improved.

Over the next year her disorder becomes worse, making it extremely difficult to walk. Finally, a neurologist diagnoses the problem, but not until permanent damage has occurred. Had the gastroenterologist warned the patient of the possible side effects of the medication or warned the PCP to watch for side effects, or had the PCP not made the erroneous assumption that the problem was due to diabetes, the medication could have been stopped when the neurological problem was still reversible.

A mistake, even a tragic one, should not be immediately equated with incompetence and gross negligence. True incompetence and gross negligence are rare but some cases do represent egregious errors. The following is an example of a flagrantly mismanaged case. A pulmonary (lung) doctor looked at a CT scan of the lungs of one of his patients and diagnosed a tumor adjacent to the main pulmonary artery of the right lung. The pulmonologist was not an expert at reading the CT scan but believed he was. Despite a report by the radiologist that stated clearly and definitively that the patient's CT scan was normal in the right lung, the pulmonologist insisted a tumor was present. The pulmonologist took the patient for bronchoscopy and did a "blind" biopsy. Tragically, it was not a tumor but a large pulmonary artery that was biopsied. The biopsy created a gaping hole in the wall of the artery. The patient bled uncontrollably and died.

This is an example of malpractice resulting from both negligence and incompetence. The pulmonologist misread the CT scan (the first error). His arrogance caused him to ignore the interpretation of the radiologist (the second error), and his disregard for caution (the third error) caused him to perform a blind rather than an open biopsy procedure (an open procedure would have revealed that there was no tumor; thus no biopsy would have been performed).

In this malpractice case, there was a disastrous outcome which resulted from a combination of arrogance, negligence, incompetence. Still, it should be kept in mind that the doctor who performed the biopsy (and directly caused the patient's death) was trying to help and save the patient's life. The intention of almost all doctors, even those who commit malpractice, is still to serve and save and care for the life of their patients. Physicians are usually correct in their judgments but they do make mistakes. Unfortunately, the mistakes can be fatal or disabling. Patients' rights to competent health care are sometimes violated. **Although negligence and incompetence do occur, they should not be confused with errors of judgment.** And it is important to realize that not all disastrous results are the result of negligence or incompetence. "Reasonable" errors of judgment often appear the same as incompetence when viewed in hindsight. After the fact, it is all to easy to discover where things went wrong and assign guilt. But in real time, providing faultless care is simply not that easy.

MEDICAL MALPRACTICE

Tee shirts were being handed out declaring a victory for a prestigious New York law firm. Caviar and champagne were flowing as freely as chips and beer at a Super Bowl Party. To paraphrase a freshman lawyer, the celebration was a company party for winning a medical malpractice case—one of the largest settlements of its kind, he said. The lawyers, he said, really did a great job of appealing to the jury's emotions rather than focusing on the facts. That's why they got such a big prize.

We live in a litigious society. Whenever someone suffers a bad outcome in any aspect of their life, there usually must be someone to blame; someone who must be punished and someone who must pay large sums of money to them (and the lawyer) for their misfortune. Medical malpractice certainly occurs, but malpractice suits have become a type of lottery with big cash prizes, mostly for lawyers.

A lawyer might tell you that whenever someone is injured or has a bad outcome, there is someone who is at fault and who can be sued. From the legal perspective this may be true, and malpractice suits are often entertained whenever a person is damaged even if no mistake has been made. On the other hand, most people who are injured because of medical mistakes are not aware of them and do not sue. It is beyond the scope of this book, and of our expertise, to recommend a fair compensation system for patients and for doctors. We can, however, state clearly that our current tort system doesn't work well for either party.

WHO CAN MAKE HEALTH CARE DECISIONS?

Competent adults have the right to accept or refuse health care. An adult is usually presumed competent, unless evidence to the contrary is obvious or becomes known. Reasons for incompetence include:
- mental illness
- developmental disability
- senility
- drunkenness
- excessive use of certain drugs

• other conditions that render the individual incapable of decision making

A surrogate decision maker is a person or persons who make a health care decision for another person (usually a minor or an adult deemed incompetent to make decisions). The laws, which vary from state to state, define who may be a surrogate decision maker. In descending order of decision-making priority, surrogate decision makers most often are:
• The patient's legal guardian
• The individual with durable power of attorney
• The patient's spouse
• The patient's adult children
• The patient's parents
• The patient's adult siblings

No surrogate decision maker can provide informed consent, if a surrogate decision maker of higher ranking has already refused to do so or if the decision is not unanimous among individuals within the same priority group. For example, if the decision makers with the highest priority for a patient are the patient's adult children, then all of them need to agree on the course of action before giving informed consent. If they do not agree, then the consent cannot be granted.

The surrogate decision maker must consider the stated wishes of the patient and abide by them in determining the course of action. Given that, surrogate decision makers are expected to make "good faith" decisions in the best interests of the patient. They also should strive to avoid any possible conflicts of interest between the patient and the decision maker.

If no surrogate is available, then the attending physician or hospital must seek a court appointed guardian to act on the patient's behalf. Also if the physician believes the surrogate decision maker's actions are not in the patient's best interests and may in fact cause the patient harm, then the physician should take appropriate measures to protect the patient. This would include seeking the advice of other surrogate decision makers or getting a court appointed legal guardian for the patient.

Minors (persons younger than 18 years), for the most part, are not allowed under state laws to make decisions about their health care. However, most states stipulate some exceptions to this general rule.

In Washington state in 1998, for example, a minor patient 14 years or older can seek and consent to medical treatment for sexually transmitted diseases or drug and alcohol abuse. Also in Washington, a minor patient can choose or refuse birth control, choose and refuse abortion, and choose to receive care during pregnancy. The rules regarding the treatment of minors differ from state to state so you need to learn about the applicable laws in your state.

Under certain circumstances, the courts can intervene in the decision-making process for the care of a minor and deny the decision of the adult guardian. If it is felt that a decision to not treat the minor would lead to irreparable harm, the court may order treatment to be administered. For example, if the parent's religious beliefs prevented potentially life saving surgery on a child, then a court could overrule the parents and order that the surgery be performed. Similar issues may apply in cases where treatment or lack thereof would injure an unborn fetus. For example, there are now medications that a pregnant woman can take which greatly reduces the chance of the fetus contracting HIV from the mother. The ethical question currently being decided by the courts is whether or not the mother can be forced to take the HIV medications during her pregnancy.

Finally, it is important to discuss your medical wishes with your doctor, family, and friends. They might be called to act upon your behalf during a medical emergency.

PATIENT RESPONSIBILITIES

Patient responsibilities are poorly defined by the legal system, but clearly, you do have an ethical responsibility to participate in your health care. Patients also have the moral responsibility to relay truthful information to their physicians. If partially true or blatantly false information is given to the doctor, a serious error in diagnosis or treatment could occur which would be entirely the patient's fault and responsibility.

Another responsibility centers on an activity which is all too common, sharing of prescribed medications. It is technically a crime to share your prescribed medications with anyone. This is especially true if the medication is a controlled substance, such as a narcotic. The consequences of sharing medications are great as the prescribed medicine might cause the other person to suffer a severe reaction and cause considerable harm to that person's health.

MEDICAL STUDIES: IS ANYONE WATCHING OUT FOR YOUR SAFETY?

Sally opened up her newspaper and read about a study involving a new medication designed to treat gastro-esophageal reflux—heartburn. She was very interested in participating but didn't know if the study was safe. So, she called the newspaper in which the advertisement appeared. They couldn't tell her anything about the study, but the medical editor recommended that she call her local hospital. The hospital informed Sally that her first step was to find out if the study had **IRB approval**. If it didn't, she probably shouldn't participate. If it did, then she would be wise to further discuss the safety of the research with her doctor and the study investigators.

IRB stands for investigational review board. It is a committee of individuals that reviews medical studies that are performed within hospitals. They serve as the patient's advocate. The board is usually composed of physicians and concerned citizens that serve as the medical watchdog for your community. Their job is to protect patients and healthy volunteers who participate in medical studies. This committee reviews both the study protocol (rules) and the informed consent. The study protocol is reviewed to ensure that the patient is not subjected to unnecessary dangers. Informed consent is a document, much like a contract, that explains to the participants the risks and benefits of joining the study. Participants are asked to sign an informed consent form when they enter a study.

If the study is dangerous or places participants at unreasonable risk, or if the study is poorly conceived, or does not create any benefit to the patient or to medical science, then the IRB will usually reject the study, thus protecting the community's medical safety.

Nevertheless, just because a study has been passed by an IRB committee does not guarantee its safety. In fact, all complications and adverse reactions must be monitored and reported to the IRB committee during the course of a study. If too many complications occur, the study may be discontinued.

Individuals are most frequently asked to participate in a study to test new medications, new medical devices, or new medical procedures. In general, most studies that pass through the IRB are valuable to medical science. They are the reason we have many of the modern advances we enjoy, such as new cancer treatments, better antibiotics, and less invasive surgical procedures. If you have a cancer not curable by traditional treatments then an experimental drug may be your only hope.

Still, individuals participating in experimental studies should take heed. Studies are being performed by companies whose motives are monetary and by doctors who may be participating in order to make extra money or receive professional recognition. Individuals often are lured into these studies by promises of free medical treatment or cash stipends. In turn, this makes patients feel obligated to continue in a study even if they are apprehensive or feel it is unsafe. For these reasons, it is important that if you participate in a study you understand how that study may affect your well-being, both now and in the future. Also, you need to know that you can quit the study at any time, and legally there can be no penalty to you if you quit.

Finally, not all studies are IRB approved. If the study is not performed in a hospital; if it is not part of a university or national study program; or if it is not being performed to obtain FDA approval, then be wary that the study may not be IRB approved. Some studies performed in doctors' offices or advertised in newspapers are not IRB approved. Put simply, **if a study is not IRB approved, there is a greater danger that it may be dangerous to your health** because the study may not meet the strict medical safety guidelines that the federal government and the local IRB committees demand.

IS YOUR PRIVACY BEING PROTECTED?

A less publicized provision of the Health Insurance Portability Act (HIPA) might have Orwellian consequences if it is not very carefully implemented. The Act instructed the Department of Health and Human Services (HHS) to develop standards for the assignment of a "Standard Unique Health Identifier" to every citizen. This identifier is intended to be confidential; however, it is to be used by both government and private health insurance payers to track and transmit all types of health information, including medical, personal and financial data. This information will be stored in a centralized "clearinghouse" and will be available to all health plans providing health benefits in the United States. HHS will impose penalties for noncompliance, misuse, or fraudulent use of this information.

Most of us want our encounters with our doctors to be kept confidential. We also want to have control over who has access to personal and financial information. Additionally, we also want to guarantee our right to have insurance coverage for certain health related matters without sacrificing our right to privacy. The provisions of the HIPA, however, jeopardizes this right to privacy. It is up to you to use your skills to protect your right to privacy. This can be accomplished by staying abreast of health related political developments and by assuming the role of an activist. You always have the power to lobby your congressional representatives and senators about these political developments and to protect your rights.

ADVANCE DIRECTIVES (PREDETERMINED GUIDELINES FOR CARE)

Advance directives are instructions given by competent individuals to their doctor and hospital defining how they would like to be treated if they develop a terminal condition. Advance directives also apply if a patient is in a permanent unconscious state or unable to give competent verbal instructions. A terminal condition is defined as an incurable and irreversible condition that would within reasonable medical judgment cause death within a reasonable period of time. In this situation, life sustaining measures would only serve to prolong the process of dying. A permanent unconscious condition also means an incurable and irreversible condition in which there is no reasonable probability of recovery from a coma or persistent vegetative state. Usually, two physicians are needed to decide if a permanent unconscious condition exists.

Both living wills and durable powers of attorney are advance directives.

- **A LIVING WILL** provides specific directions as to what type of medical treatment you want or do not want in the event you become incompetent.
- **A DURABLE POWER OF ATTORNEY** appoints someone else to make decisions and give instruction in the event that your become incompetent.

In 1991, the national Patient Self-Determination Act was passed requiring nursing homes, hospitals, and health plans to ask patients if they had an advanced directive and to incorporate these directives into the patient's medical records. Advance directives do not have to be permanent documents, and can be revoked by the patient in writing, or in some states even orally. If family members, doctors, or any other interested persons do not agree with the advance directive, they must petition the court to have it overturned. If the court doesn't do this, then the doctor can follow the advance directive despite the family's contrary wishes.

To prevent the courts from becoming involved, you should candidly discuss your wishes with your family and surrogate decision makers to try to make them understand and accept your wishes and personal choices.

The problems with advance directives revolve around unanticipated circumstances that might be the subject of varying interpretations. Most living will documents contain language about limiting "extraordinary measures" to prolong life. The limitations an advance directive will often place on health care treatments usually focus on life support technology, which includes:

- intubation and ventilator support
- dialysis
- temporary pacemakers
- cardiopulmonary resuscitation (CPR)
- medications (other than those to relieve pain)
- artificial nutrition and hydration
- defibrillation (shocking the heart with an electric current to restart the heart)

Exercise 19-1 will assist you in thinking through some of the treatment issues we have discussed in this chapter. We encourage you to share this exercise with both your surrogate decision maker(s) and your doctor. Advance directive forms are usually available at hospitals, libraries, or office supply stores.

THE RIGHT TO DIE

If the principles of personal autonomy are strictly applied—that one always has the right of free choice as long as no harm comes to others—then suicide should be an option to those competent individuals who choose it. This, however, is in direct contrast with the spirit of federal and state laws which attempt to preserve life. In fact, in the past, suicide was a crime in many states.

Euthanasia, a term first used in 1869, means "the good death or easy and happy death." There are several different forms of euthanasia.

With **VOLUNTARY EUTHANASIA,** the sufferer asks for measures to be taken to end his or her life. Under this form, the physician would take an active role in ending the patient's life.

Voluntary euthanasia incorporates the current call by some in our country for physician assisted suicide. This issue is being discussed both at the medical and legal levels. Some people believe that laws which prohibit physicians from prescribing life ending medications to competent adults who wish to hasten the process of their death are unconstitutional because they violate the 14th Amendment (no person can be denied "life, liberty, or property without due process of law"). Other people believe it is discriminatory to refuse terminally ill patients the right to terminate with medications their lives when other dying patients can refuse life sustaining medical treatment.

Consequently, the U.S. legal system is being confronted by these and other issues. However, at the time of this writing, no physician in this country can legally assist a patient in voluntary euthanasia. Only the Northern Territory of Australia legally allows voluntary euthanasia. The Netherlands has permissive laws which allow doctors to help patients die under certain conditions, but voluntary euthanasia is technically illegal in that country.

PASSIVE EUTHANASIA implies the deliberate withholding of treatment thereby ending the patient's life. This form of euthanasia gets carried out through the use of advance directives.

COMPULSORY EUTHANASIA means that a society or a person acting on authority gives instructions to terminate the life of a person who cannot express his or her wishes. This form of euthanasia should not be practiced by anyone anywhere.

There are several issues to contemplate when discussing euthanasia. First, is refusing treatment for a severe illness suicide or is it just the hastening of a natural death? Refusing treatment for bacterial meningitis, which when untreated is nearly 100 percent fatal, might or might not be different from actively taking a deadly poison. Second, do patients need to be classified as "terminal" in the strictest sense of the word before being allowed to terminate their life? Patients can have severely debilitating diseases, which can result in chronic pain and dependency, and still be able to live a normal life span with the disease. However, some of these patients may believe that their lives have little or no "quality" and would prefer to die early.

Third, should physicians play a role in euthanasia? Patients wanting to end their life often would rather be given a substance that can be used under the auspices of their physician. This provides them with a sense of security that the task will be done properly and thought-fully. However, the physician plays a role in the death of a patient in a marked divergence from the traditional role as a healer. Does this present a conflict of interest for the doctor?

CONCLUSIONS

The technology that improves and lengthens our lives also creates many questions about how that technology should be used. There are no right or wrong answers, only opinions. In the perfect world, your personal choices would determine your own course of action. After all, what is right for you might not be right for another and vice versa. But as we all know, society, whether rightfully or not, plays a role in all of our choices.

EXERCISE 19-1

Health Care Decisions and Advance Directives

It is in your best interest to answer the following questions as truthfully as possible, no matter how painful it may be to you. You should share your answers with the individual(s) who will act as your surrogate decision-maker(s) in the event that you are not mentally competent to make your own decisions. You will also want to discuss your responses with your primary care doctor and, as warranted, with any specialists from which you seek care.

1. Do you want to know the truth about your condition?
   Always   Sometimes   Never

Explain _____

_____

_____

2. Do you want to be involved in making decisions regarding your health care treatment?
   Always   Sometimes   Never

Explain _____

_____

_____

3. Under what physical or mental limitations do you anticipate not being able to participate in the decision-making process?

_____

_____

4. Do you want to be an organ donor when you die? Yes   No

If yes, explain _____

_____

_____

5. During a terminal illness, where do you prefer to receive care and why:
   In the comfort of your own home?   In a hospice facility?
   In a skilled nursing facility?   In a hospital?

Explain _____

EXERCISE 19-1

Health Care Decisions and Advance Directives
(cont.)

6. If your health condition or family situation required it, how would you feel about being placed in a nursing home?

Explain _____

_____

_____

7. Do you want your financial situation taken into account when your treatment decisions are made?

Explain _____

_____

_____

8. Do you think life-sustaining measures should be used:
   If you have a terminal illness?
   If you are in a coma?
   If you suffer from an irreversible chronic disease, such as Alzheimer's?

Explain _____

_____

_____

9. When would you not want the following medical procedures?

Mechanical breathing (respirator) Kidney dialysis
Cardio-pulmonary resuscitation   Pain relief medication
   (CPR)   Chemotherapy or radiation
                                      therapy
Artificial nutrition and hydration Being placed in an intensive
   (feeding tubes)   care unit
Antibiotics   Surgery
Blood transfusion

Explain _____

_____

_____

Health Care Decisions and Advance Directives
(cont.)

10. In regards to your medical treatment, what do the following phrases mean to you:

Letting nature take its course

Quality of life

Living as long as possible

Being independent

Being comfortable and pain free

A lingering death

Being mentally aware and competent

Being able to spend time with family or friends

Being able to incorporate spiritual beliefs and traditions

Explain _____

_____

_____

_____

_____

_____

_____

_____

_____

_____

_____

_____

_____

_____

_____

_____

_____

_____

_____

Becoming Your Own Best Patient Advocate

Becoming **your own best patient advocate** requires time, energy, and endurance. The reward for your effort, however, is better health, a better quality of life, and the sense that you are working with your doctor to help influence the direction of your care. It is analogous to riding a canoe down the rapids of a river. Would you prefer to travel with or without a paddle? With or without a guide?

The following stories illustrate the differences between the passive and the proactive patient.

CLUELESS

Two women were sharing a room in the hospital. Both suffered from congestive heart failure, a condition where the lungs fill up with water and breathing becomes difficult. This is caused when the heart muscle is damaged and it pumps the blood too weakly to maintain normal circulation.

The day before their hospitalization, both women became short of breath and needed to be seen in the emergency room.

Shirley's doctor immediately recognized she was in congestive heart failure (CHF) and restricted her fluids, salt intake, and gave her diuretics (water pills).

In contrast, Mildred's doctor came in and did not initially appreciate that she was in congestive heart failure. He started an IV and gave her more fluids, which actually caused her to slip further into congestive heart failure. She became so bad that she started having increasing chest pain and suffered angina (lack of oxygen to the heart). Upon recognizing his error, Mildred's doctor prescribed medications to treat her CHF. No permanent damage was done but the extra fluids had put Mildred's already weak heart at risk.

That next morning the two women were in their rooms discussing their illnesses and their doctors. Mildred expounded on how brilliant and wonderful her doctor was. "He pulled me out from the jaws of death," she proudly declared, never knowing that he had actually pushed her deeper into her predicament.

Shirley naively and sheepishly responded. "Maybe I should change doctors. I'm not sure that my doctor is as good as yours or could save my life if I became that ill. I came into the hospital and was feeling better within 6 hours. I must not be as sick as you. What's the name of your doctor? I should keep him in mind if I ever really get ill."

One problem is that neither patient had a clue about the care their doctors had delivered. Shirley thought her doctor was bad when he had delivered excellent care. Mildred thought her doctor was excellent when he had initially delivered poor care. Both left the hospital with incorrect impressions as to the care that they had received.

People are often clueless about the care they receive. This can restrict the quality of their life and prove dangerous to their health. Contrast these two patients' passive approach to the approach taken by Delores in the next story.

CREATING YOUR OWN MEDICAL MIRACLE

When you spoke to Delores you couldn't help but notice that her attractive face was periodically contorted by violent muscular contractions called tics. They began in 1979 at age 50 as gentle twitches of the eye when she was tired or stressed. With time they grew more intense, and the twitches became spasms, and the spasms became violent contractions. They soon were brought on by almost any sudden movement of the facial muscles, especially smiling or laughing. The spasms created no physical discomfort, but Delores was painfully aware of her deformity. She was so self conscious "of those awful and humiliating contractions" that she tried not to smile.

Initially, the doctors diagnosed the spasms as being caused by stress. Her 50th year had been difficult. So the diagnosis made sense to her. She learned to reduce her stress. But even during the calmest and most harmonious years to follow, she was still plagued by spasms. Her primary care doctor insisted that the problem was stress related, but she was no longer stressed and the symptoms were worse than ever. In 1984, five years after the initial diagnosis, Delores decided it was time to take matters into her own hands and seek a second opinion.

She has diagnosed by an ophthalmologist as having hemifacial spasm. The cause of her spasms was idiopathic (unknown). Although a CT scan did reveal some prominent vessels located near her left seventh cranial nerve (the nerve that controls facial movement) these vessels were believed to be incidental and not causing the symptoms. To control the spasms she received botulism toxin injections in the region surrounding her affected left eye. These injections controlled the severity but did not cure the spasms. At first the injections were given once every nine months and yielded excellent control. But over time the frequency of injections increased while symptomatic relief diminished. She grew worried about the effect the medications would have on her body. She had learned about patients whose faces became paralyzed and who developed resistant antibodies to the injections.

For 10 years she endured the injections. Although she was grateful for the relief they offered she still desired a more permanent cure. She asked her doctors for additional suggestions and was told that she "should be happy with the relief she was experiencing with the injections." For Delores, this was not acceptable.

She joined a national support organization of individuals with similar problems. At first, she worried that she might discover individuals whose symptoms began like hers but grew more and more crippling. She overcame that fear and to her encouragement instead learned of a women who had been cured by an operation performed by a doctor in Pittsburgh.

Delores asked her doctors about the treatments. Again they told her she was doing well and they felt surgery was too risky. They had drawn this conclusion without full knowledge of this particular doctor's experience or new techniques.

On her own Delores continued to research cures other than botulism toxin. Delores went to the local hospital library and with the help of the hospital librarian did a literature review (using MEDLINE and the Internet). The review included articles by the Pittsburgh doctor. In the articles Delores discovered that one of the causes of hemifacial spasms is abnormal blood vessels irritating the facial nerve. This doctor in Pittsburgh had developed a surgical procedure in which he could cure patients by treating these abnormal blood vessels. At that point, Delores recalled she had been told years earlier that she had abnormal vessels near her facial nerve. Her research also revealed that she could further diagnose this condition by an MRI with vascular imaging study.

Delores returned to her family practice physician fortified with this knowledge. Although he was skeptical of the usefulness of the tests, because of Delores' insistence he ordered the MRI. The MRI revealed three abnormal vessels winding around and likely irritating the facial nerve. She met with the radiologist who reviewed the MRI films with her. Delores asked him for his opinion and advice. After reviewing the pertinent medical journal articles (she had brought them with her) he called the referring family practice doctor and reported that Delores should be an excellent candidate for the surgery. Privately, he also encouraged Delores to "go for it." She called the doctor in Pittsburgh who told her to send the films. After reviewing the images he agreed with the findings and recommended surgery. She called her insurance company to get prior approval for the operation. Because she was fee-for-service and not part of a more restrictive HMO or managed care program, they informed her that insurance would cover most of the expenses.

When Delores came back to visit her doctors one month after the surgery, her 67-year-old face was beaming with a smile that revealed her joy and elation. "My life has been changed. I am so happy I was persistent and investigated cures other than that botulism toxin. Thank you. I am grateful to the doctors who believed in me and encouraged and helped me in my long journey to be cured."

Delores' story is about creating medical miracles. Some miracles just happen. Others require assistance. Today, Delores is cured and is assisting others to achieve their own miraculous cures. Delores' journey took 15 years and it was not easy. She had to learn by trial and error.

Delores didn't have a book to assist her through her medical journey. Many of the lessons discussed within this book including how and when to be persistent, when to ask for help, who to trust, and most importantly, how to help yourself, are lessons Delores had to learn on her own.

It is the hope of the authors that by applying the information and lessons within this book, you can make your own medical miracle a reality.

To get the care you deserve, you need to:
1. Learn how to communicate effectively with your doctor
2. Get prepared and organized for your appointment
3. Take responsibility for ensuring that you are receiving excellent care
4. Select an insurance plan that meets your medical needs
5. Understand and protect your medical rights

PATIENTS' BILL OF RIGHTS
We first introduced these patient rights in Chapter 14, but we feel they bear repeating. At a minimum, patients should expect and be entitled to the following:

PATIENTS SHOULD...
- Be informed of all their medical options
- Have the right to choose the doctor they want (including specialists) in order to get the care they need
- Have medical decisions made by medical experts not insurance companies, managed care companies, or hospital administrators
- Have access to emergency room care wherever and whenever it is needed
- Have all medical records kept confidential
- Be guaranteed quality care

References and Recommended Readings

ALTERNATIVE AND CONVENTIONAL MEDICAL CARE

Alternative Medicine compiled by the Burton Goldberg Group

The American Medical Association's Guide to Your Family's Symptoms by Charles B. Clayman and Raymond H. Curry

Beyond Prozac by Michael Norden

A Cancer Survivor's Almanac by the National Coalition for Cancer Survivorship

Consumer's Medical Desk Reference by Charles B. Inlander of the People's Medical Society

Dr. Dean Ornish's Program for Reversing Heart Disease by Dean Ornish

Enter the Zone by Barry Sears

Eight Weeks to Optimal Health by Andrew Weil

Examining Your Doctor by Timothy B. McCall

The Doctor's Book of Home Remedies edited by Debora Tkac

Dr. Koop's Self Care Advisor by C. Everett Koop

The Medical Advisor: The Complete Guide to Alternative and Conventional Treatments by the editors of TimeLife Books

Mayo Clinic Family Health Book edited by David E. Larson

Optimal Wellness by Ralph Golan

Physician's Desk Reference by Medical Economics Data

Power Sleep by James Maas

Prepare for Surgery, Heal Faster by Peggy Huddleston

Harrison's Principles of Internal Medicine by Anthony Fauci

Principles of Surgery by Seymour I. Schwartz

MIND-BODY APPROACHES TO MEDICINE

Anatomy of an Illness by Norman Cousins

The Book of Job translated by Steven Mitchell

Healing and the Mind by Bill Moyers

Love, Medicine and Miracles by Bernie S. Siegel

Love is Letting Go of Fear by Gerald Jampolsky

Loving Each Other and Living, Loving and Learning by Leo Buscaglia

Man's Search for Meaning by Viktor E. Frankl

On Death and Dying by Elisabeth Kubler-Ross

Unlimited Power and *Personal Power* by Anthony Robbins

The Road Less Traveled by Scott Peck

Siddhartha by Hermann Hesse

Unconditional Life: Discovering the Power to Fulfill Your Dreams by Deepak Chopra

You'll See It When You Believe It by Wayne Dyer

HEALTH INFORMATION SOURCES

Consumer's Guide to Free Medical Information by Phone and Mail by Arthur Winter and Ruth Winter

Health Online by Tom Feruson

Legal Documents and Forms for Medicine by EZ Legal Forms

MEDICAL HISTORY AND CURRENT EVENTS

Medicine: An Illustrated History by Albert Lyons and R. Joseph Petrucelli

Speak Now or Forever Rest in Peace by Gordon Miller

Types of Providers and Therapies

SPECIALTIES—TRADITIONAL MEDICINE

ALLOPATHIC MEDICINE (TRADITIONAL WESTERN MEDICINE, M.D.): Allopathy is the traditional Western medicine whose healing philosophy is founded on scientific principles. Illnesses are treated with medications that produce effects which are antagonistic to the cause of the disease. Implicit in this approach is the notion that active intervention by the physician is necessary. Allopathic medicine is the dominant form of medicine practiced in the United States today. Allopathic doctors complete medical school and earn the degree Doctor of Medicine (M.D.). For most of us, allopathic doctors are the ones that we have the most contact with throughout our lives.

ALLERGY & IMMUNOLOGY: subspecialty of either Internal Medicine or Pediatrics that deals with the diagnosis and treatment of allergic and related disorders including asthma, food allergies, etc., and other rarer conditions that involve the immune system.

ANESTHESIOLOGY: specialty that deals with the administration of medications to produce numbness or induce "unconsciousness" so that painful procedures, such as surgery, can be performed. Some anesthesiologists specialize in the management of chronic pain as well as in critical care medicine.

CARDIOLOGY: subspecialty of Internal Medicine or Pediatrics that diagnoses and treats problems with the heart and circulatory system.

CARDIOTHORACIC SURGERY: subspecialty of General Surgery that diagnoses and treats surgical problems in the chest cavity including the heart, lungs, and blood vessels. These physicians routinely perform coronary artery bypass surgery and repair aneurysms.

DERMATOLOGY: specialty that diagnoses and treats skin ailments.

EMERGENCY MEDICINE: specialty that concentrates on the diagnosis and management of acute problems, such as infections, abdominal or chest pain, fractures, etc., usually in a hospital Emergency Room or acute-care walk-in clinic.

ENDOCRINOLOGY: subspecialty area of Internal Medicine or Pediatrics that diagnoses and treats glandular/hormonal problems. These physicians routinely treat diabetes, and thyroid and pituitary problems, and may treat some menstrual and sexual development disorders.

GASTROENTEROLOGY: subspecialty area of Internal Medicine or Pediatrics that diagnoses and treats problems of the digestive system including the esophagus, stomach, intestines, gall bladder, liver, and pancreas.

GERIATRICS: subspecialty of Internal Medicine that concentrates on the medical problems seen in the elderly.

HAND SURGERY: subspecialty of either Orthopedics or Plastic Surgery limited to treating disorders of the hand.

HEMATOLOGY (& ONCOLOGY): subspecialty area of either Internal Medicine or Pediatrics that diagnoses and treats problems with the blood and blood forming elements including anemia; these physicians are usually trained in the treatment of cancer as well.

INFECTIOUS DISEASE: subspecialty of Internal Medicine or Pediatrics that concentrates on the diagnosis and treatment of infections including those caused by bacteria, viruses, fungi, and parasites. These are the physicians who usually manage patients with AIDS.

INTERNAL MEDICINE: an "internist" (*note:* not an "intern") is trained to diagnose and treat diseases that affect adults. Medical sub-specialists are trained as internists then receive additional training in the sub-specialty area (for example, cardiology).

MAXILLOFACIAL SURGERY: subspecialty area of dentistry that deals with the diagnosis and treatment of surgical problems affecting the mouth and the jaw.

NEONATOLOGY: subspecialty of pediatrics that diagnoses and treats problems in newborn infants including premature birth.

NEPHROLOGY: subspecialty of Internal Medicine or Pediatrics concerning itself with the diagnosis and treatment of diseases affecting the kidney.

NEUROLOGY: specialty that treats disorders affecting the brain, spinal cord, and peripheral nerves; these doctors routinely treat strokes and epilepsy.

NEUROSURGERY: surgical subspecialty that treats disorders of the brain, spinal cord, and peripheral nervous system.

OBSTETRICS (& GYNECOLOGY): specialty that delivers babies, diagnoses and manages pregnancy as well as the disorders that affect the female genital tract. Some of these physicians specialize in fertility problems.

ONCOLOGY: subspecialty of Internal Medicine dealing with the diagnosis and treatment of cancer.

OPTHALMOLOGY: subspecialty that does both medical and surgical treatment of eye diseases. These doctors treat glaucoma and often do cataract surgery.

ORTHOPEDIC SURGERY: surgical subspecialty that treats bone, joint, tendon, and other musculoskeletal soft tissue disorders, including joint replacement surgery and the setting of fractures.

OTORHINOLARYNGOLOGY (ENT): surgical subspecialty for the diagnosis and treatment of disorders that affect the ear, nose, and throat.

PATHOLOGY: specialty that examines bodily tissues and fluids to aid other physicians in diagnosing their patients. Pathologists are the doctors who interpret biopsies, perform autopsies, and supervise hospital laboratories.

PEDIATRICS (PEDIATRICIAN): specialty that deals with children from birth to young adulthood.

PHYSICAL MEDICINE (PHYSIATRIST): specialty that evaluates and treats physical impairments, usually which result from diseases of the nervous or musculoskeletal system, in order to help a person maximize their physical function and maintain independence. These physicians usually participate in the rehabilitation of stroke victims.

PODIATRY: An area of medical practice that deals with disorders and treatments of the foot and lower leg. Podiatrists are not trained as classic allopathic M.D.s but rather complete four years of school and a residency which deal with medical and surgical management of foot disorders. Podiatric practice overlaps with orthopedic physicians.

PSYCHIATRY (PSYCHIATRIST): specialty that treats mental disorders such as depression, mania, and schizophrenia.

PULMONARY MEDICINE (PULMONOLOGIST): subspecialty of Internal Medicine that deals with disorders of the lung and bronchial tree including asthma, chronic bronchitis, emphysema, and pneumonia. Often, these physicians also specialize in managing patients in intensive care units in hospitals.

RADIOLOGY (RADIOLOGIST): specialty that interprets x-rays and other technologies including ultrasound and MRI, which image the internal structure of the body. A subspecialty of radiology is interventional radiology where catheters are used with x-ray guidance to diagnose and treat an expanding range of illness without using surgery.

PLASTIC SURGERY: subspecialty of general surgery in which a variety of surgical techniques are used to improve appearance and function. These physicians can treat congenital deformities or repair the scars of burn victims.

RHEUMATOLOGY (RHEUMATOLOGIST): subspecialty of Internal Medicine that deals with the medical treatment of arthritis, bone, muscle and tendon problems, and disorders of the immune system called autoimmune diseases. These physicians treat osteoarthritis, osteoporosis, rheumatoid arthritis, and lupus.

UROLOGY (UROLOGIST): surgical subspecialty that diagnoses and surgically treats disorders of the kidney, urinary system including the bladder, as well as male reproductive problems including impotence.

VASCULAR SURGERY: surgical subspecialty that treats disorders of blood vessels, excluding those in the heart, lungs, or brain.

OTHER TYPES OF PROVIDERS
MIDWIFE: a person trained in the supervision, care, and advice to women during pregnancy, labor, and the postpartum period and trained to conduct deliveries without supervision.

NURSE PRACTITIONER: a registered nurse, with a masters degree, who has completed an advanced education and clinical training program in a health care specialty, such as a geriatric nurse practitioner, nurse anesthetist, nurse mid-wife, etc. A nurse practitioner functions independently from physicians.

PHYSICIAN ASSISTANT: a health professional who has completed a two-year physician assistant training program, practices medicine under the supervision of a physician, and can perform the tasks delegated by the supervising physician.

PSYCHOLOGIST: a health professional that has training in psychological theory and counseling. Those with a bachelor's or master's degree in psychology can provide counseling services. Clinical Psychologists have a doctoral degree, and have completed original research and a year of internship.

SPECIALTIES—ALTERNATIVE MEDICINE

Usually you are not limited to one type of treatment. There are many alternatives available. No matter which type of treatment you choose, you will be better served by understanding the philosophy and goals that the different treatments offer. A brief description of the different types of treatments is listed below.

ACUPUNCTURE: This is an ancient Chinese healing art. It uses needles to balance the flow of vital energy, chi, in the body in order to heal disease and promote health. These needles are believed to block pain pathways in order to achieve relief or alter muscle and nerve function.

AYURVEDIC *(i-a-vedic)* **MEDICINE:** Ayurvedic medicine originated in India; its approach is based upon the ancient Hindu art of medicine. The core belief is that each individual has a specific body type and that disease is the result of an imbalance in the body's energy and habits. By altering diet and lifestyle and through herbal/medical/ spiritual avenues, the body can be healed. Dr. Deepak Chopra's books help explain this medical philosophy.

HERBAL MEDICINE: An alternative healing art that uses plants instead of synthetic compounds (medicines), to prevent and treat disease. The herbalist will look for the cause of the disease then will recommend the missing nutritional elements and herbs that are needed to strengthen your body. This is a growing practice in the United States today. Most herbalists seek training from other herbalists.

Herbology is considered by many to be the natural approach to medical treatment. As an interesting note, modern pharmacology is based upon this treatment method. Most drugs used today are typically the synthetic derivatives of the curative parts of natural plants. The best example is aspirin. It is a synthetic derivative of salicin, derived from willow bark.

HOLISTIC MEDICINE: This represents a philosophical approach to patient care in which the physical, mental, and social factors in the patient's condition are all taken into consideration rather than just focusing on the diagnosed disease. Any physician with any type of training can be a holistic practitioner.

HOMEOPATHY: a system of medical treatment based on the theory that "like cures like." Substances, which in high doses produce similar symptoms as a given disease, are given to the patient in very low doses in order to treat the disease. For example, ipecac (which is used medically to induce vomiting) is given in extremely small doses by a homeopathic doctor to treat vomiting. Homeopathic remedies are prepared by progressively diluting substances and vigorously shaking the solutions to potentiate their action. The final remedy theoretically may contain none of the original substance; just the water that was used in the preparation process.

MANIPULATIVE THERAPIES: Techniques that use manual movement of the musculoskeletal system to relieve and treat pain and disease. Osteopathy and Chiropractic are practiced by individuals who have been awarded a Doctorate in the particular specialty. The practitioners of the other techniques have received specialized training in the particular area. These techniques include:

Acupressure: Fingertips are used to stimulate "meridians" which allows for the flow of "chi" (life force) to be even. Acupressure is a simpler, easier-to-use system that evolved from acupuncture. It is primarily used on the ears, hands, and feet, which have been determined to be connected to the different organs and systems of the body.

Chiropractic: This therapy emphasizes manipulation of the spine as a method to restore health. The therapy in most traditional form does not use medication but does use heat, ultrasound, and other topical modalities.

Osteopathy: An osteopath is an allopathic physician who holds the essential belief that there is a relationship between disease and the structure of the body. They use the same techniques as M.D.s in diagnosing and treating disease, but they also use manipulative therapy to treat disease, particularly musculoskeletal pain problems. Outside of manipulative techniques, their medical training is identical to that of an M.D.

MASSAGE: This therapy is a modality in which hard manipulation of the body is used to relieve pain, improve circulation, and impart relaxation. There are several types of massage therapy in use today.

Swedish: This is the most common and widely practiced.

Shiatsu: A Japanese method in which pressure is exerted in specific "meridians" to improve "Chi" (energy).

Rolfing: This uses very deep massage to improve posture and to relax various groups of muscles.

Reflexology: Certain areas of the feet which correspond to other parts of the body are stimulated.

NATUROPATHY: This is a system of medicine that relies on the use of only "natural" substances for the treatment of disease, rather than synthetic drugs. A basic premise is that the body has the inherent ability not only to heal itself and restore health, but also to ward off disease. The naturopath attempts to remove unnatural substances that interfere with the body's ability to heal itself and which are at the root of most illnesses. It uses botanical medicines, containing multiple chemicals from one or more plants, to augment the body's healing capacity.

Prevention

Change your habits and you change your health.

The best treatment is prevention. Listed below are 12 of the most important life habits. To practice effective preventive medicine apply these positive lifestyle changes.

Do not smoke or chew tobacco

Get regular exercise

Eat in moderation and create a diet that fits your body chemistry

Maintain a realistic and healthy weight

Drink alcohol in moderation or don't drink at all. Never drink and drive.

Be alert and practice basic safety, such as remembering to buckle your seatbelt, using child safety seats, and wearing a bike helmet. Also, accident-proof your house to prevent accidents and falls.

Reduce uv exposure. Restrict your time in the sun during the peak hours of 11 A.M. to 2 P.M. If you must be in the sun during peak hours, wear a sunscreen with an spf of at least 15–30 and wear a hat. Do not use tanning booths.

Avoid environmental toxins, pesticides, and harmful chemicals

Practice stress reduction. Keep your blood pressure in a healthy range

Take good care of your teeth

Avoid excess and harmful mixtures of vitamins, medications, and supplements

Perform the recommended preventive screening exams

WOMEN

Test	Age	Frequency
General health exams	Over 20	Every 3 years
	Over 40	Every year
Cholesterol Test	Over 20	Every 5 years
Pap Test & Pelvic Exam	18 and over	Annually, or after 3 normal pap smears (less frequently at the discretion of your physician)
Self Breast Exam	20 and over	Monthly
Mammography	35–39	Baseline
	40–49	Every 1–2 years
	50 and over	Annually
Digital Rectal Exam	Over 40	Annually
Stool Blood Test	Over 50	Annually
Sigmoidoscopy	50 and over	Every 3–5 years

MEN

Test	Age	Frequency
General health exams	Over 20	Every 3 years
	Over 40	Annually
Cholesterol Test	Over 20	Every 5 years
Digital Rectal Exam	Over 40	Annually
Stool Blood Test	Over 50	Annually
Sigmoidoscopy	50 and over	Every 3–5 years
Prostate Exam	50 and over	Annually
PSA Test	50 and over	Annually

Index

To the Reader

Getting the Best From Your Doctor is designed to help you find your way through the unsettled and frustrating medical maze. It is the authors' goal to empower patients through education and communication skills. This book is intended to teach you how to take charge of your medical care and well being.

Please share with us your comments about the book. Are there any medical experiences you think we should know about? Is there a subject about which you would like to learn more?

To share your stories and comments, please write to us at:

Alan Schwartz, Richard Jimenez, Tracy Myers, Andrew Solomon
Power Patient Advocates
P.O. Box 1195
Lynnwood, WA 98046-1195